MEN'S HEALTH ADVISOR 1994

MEN'S HEALTH ADVISOR 1994

EDITED BY
MICHAEL LAFAVORE

Men's Health Magazine

Rodale Press, Emmaus, Pennsylvania

ISBN 0–87596–199–1 hardcover
ISSN 1060–9407

  6 8 10 9 7 5   hardcover

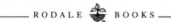

Contributors to
Men's Health Advisor 1994

EXECUTIVE EDITOR, *Men's Health* Magazine: Michael Lafavore

EDITORIAL DIRECTOR, *Men's Health* Books: Russell Wild

GROUP VICE-PRESIDENT: Mark Bricklin

PROJECT COORDINATOR: Dominick Bosco

BOOK DESIGNERS: Alfred Zelcer, Acey Lee

COVER DESIGNER: Acey Lee

COVER PHOTOGRAPHER: David Vance

ILLUSTRATOR: Hal Mayforth

BOOK LAYOUT: Ayers/Johanek Publication Design

MANAGING EDITOR, *Men's Health* Magazine: Steven Slon

RESEARCH EDITOR, *Men's Health* Magazine: Melissa Gotthardt

OFFICE STAFF, *Men's Health* Books: Julie Kehs, Roberta Mulliner, Mary Lou Stephen

OFFICE MANAGER, *Men's Health* Magazine: Susan Campbell

Contents

8 BOD LIKE A ROCK

9 TAKING CARE OF BUSINESS

10 ASK *MEN'S HEALTH*

Introduction

THE RULES
WE WRITE BY

There's no shortage of health information out there. In fact, there's probably too much of it, at least too much from the wrong sources. The newspapers delight in jumping all over every health scare that comes down the pipeline. Their reporters may not understand the issue very well, but that never seems to stop them from writing. The television news shows can be even worse. At least once a week, along about 10:00 P.M., you can expect a 30-second teaser that goes something like "NEW CANCER SCARE IN YOUR FOOD SUPPLY! IS YOUR FAMILY AT RISK? MORE AT 11."

Anyone who pays much attention to that sort of thing can't be blamed for saying something like "Everything is bad for you. I'm not even going to try to stay healthy, because something or other is going to get me anyway." And in fact, I hear one version or another of that statement far too often these days.

Since this is the *Men's Health Advisor*, and you can reasonably expect that a book by that title is going to offer you some health advice, I thought I'd explain a few of the ground rules that the writers and I used when we put this book together. Here they are.

1. Everything isn't bad for you. In fact, a lot of things are very good for you, and many of those that are bad are bad for you only if you overdo them.

2. You are in charge of your health. The lifestyle choices you make are far more important than the uncontrollable threats that the news media like to report on. In fact, research shows you can add 15 years to your life just by taking charge of some key life-shortening behaviors.

3. Change isn't easy. We don't preach, and we don't wag fingers. We know from our own experience that bad habits practiced over decades aren't broken in days. The best way to make lifestyle changes stick is to take them one at a time, phase them in gradually and set reasonable goals. You can do it.

4. Good health isn't just the absence of illness. If you take good care of yourself, you can expect to feel and look great. You can expect to have lots of energy and vitality. You can expect to enjoy life not only longer but more fully.

So turn off the television, tuck that newspaper into the recycling bin, and check out the practical and useful health information between these covers.

Michael Lafavore
Executive Editor
Men's Health Magazine

Part 1

HOW A MAN
STAYS YOUNG

Break Free of Your Rut!
Are you sleepwalking through life?
Has a dull routine taken control of your being?
Here are 29 ways to shake up and wake up your life.

● ● ● ● ● ● ● ● ● ● ● ● ● ● ● ● ● ●

LET'S START WITH A QUESTION: How did you spend the past five Saturday nights? If you can't remember, join the crowd. According to Sidney B. Simon, Ed.D., retired professor of psychological education at the University of Massachusetts, most people have trouble distinguishing one weekend from another, because quite simply, nothing memorable happened.

"What was possible for you to have done instead?" asks Dr. Simon, who writes and lectures on how to make life richer through change. "Why didn't you do something that would have been more interesting?" If your answer is that you couldn't think of anything better to do, or that you just didn't feel like trying something different, you may be suffering from a very common dilemma: You're stuck in a rut.

Almost everybody slides into a comfortable but boring track at one time or another. Ruts start out innocently enough: Often they're simple routines that meet a real need for stability and consistency in a chaotic and unpredictable world. We take the same route to work because it's the fastest or most trouble-free. We buy the same suit in three different colors so that we can look acceptable without giving it a moment's thought. We habitually watch TV after dinner because it makes us feel comfortable and relaxed after a nerve-shredding day at work.

Eventually, however, routines can acquire a life of their own. Designed to help us maintain control, they begin to *take* control, until very little is left to chance and nothing seems new anymore.

ARE YOU A POD PERSON?

"A rut is a routine taken too far," says Ken Druck, Ph.D., an executive consultant and an expert on the Type A personality. "There's such a thing as too much predictability and consistency."

A rut is when you order the same meal at the same Italian restaurant every Friday. It's when you take your wife and kids for granted and develop a verbal shorthand with them, so you never really talk. It's when you get so good at your job that you could do it in a coma. It's when you take the same vacation to the same cabin every year. It's when you avoid emotional or physical chances, make love perfunctorily, never seek out new friends or call old ones for fear that you'll have nothing to say. It's when you always wear boxer shorts. It's when the real you seems to have been replaced by a pod person from *Invasion of the Body Snatchers*.

"When you're in a rut, you fail to update the ways you think and live, even if your needs have changed," says Salvatore Maddi, Ph.D., professor of psychology at the

University of California, Irvine, and president of the Hardiness Institute, a psychological consulting firm. "If you're no longer learning from new experiences or growing as a person, it means you're missing out on a big part of life."

When you break free of circumscribing habits, you reap a wide range of benefits. You spur your mind to think in new ways; you become more energetic, more creative and better able to solve problems. The net effect is that you're happier—and often more successful. Best of all, the process begins with small changes. The experts say there's no need to sell all your possessions and move to Bali. Instead, minor adjustments in the ways you think, behave and even dress are all it takes to add spice to life. Not only is that easier than hopping a Java-bound flight on Air Garuda, it's also less expensive.

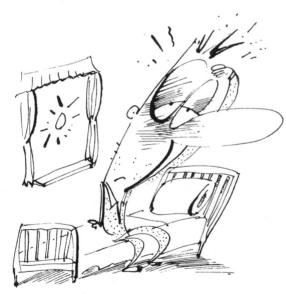

Sleep on the Wagon

It's so late even Conan O'Brien is sound asleep somewhere, while you're still tossing and turning. But don't bother getting up to fix yourself a drink.

Drinking alcohol disturbs sleep rather than helping it, says Landgrave Smith, Ph.D., assistant professor at the University of Oklahoma Health Sciences Center. "Alcohol makes you spend less time in deep sleep and more time in light sleep and dreaming, so you won't feel rested the next day anyway," he explains. Better to figure out what's keeping you awake. Anxiety, depression, noise and discomfort are common culprits. "Attack the problem," Dr. Smith says, "not the symptom. If you treat the anxiety, for example, the sleep disturbance will fade away."

RUT PATROL

Before you can even begin to climb out of a rut, you need to be aware that you're in one. There's an element of embarrassment in this. No man likes to admit his life is anything less than enviable. However, recognizing a rut for what it is is a sign of mental strength. "It means you're in touch with your innate desire to grow," says Neil Fiore, Ph.D., a Berkeley, California, psychologist and author of *The Now Habit.* "It's a sign that you're not being challenged, that you have reached a certain level of competence and are moving toward greater fulfillment."

The major symptom is boredom, a squalid sense of sameness, which it's possible to experience even when the trappings of your life are exciting or demanding. Boredom is a form of stress, says Dr. Maddi. But even if you're not aware of being bored, if you're in a rut you'll feel a twinge of malaise at some point just about every day. That point is often first thing in the morning. If you generally don't look forward to the day ahead, it may be time to start making a few changes.

To do it, there are some general principles that apply no matter what area of life you seem to be stuck in.

The first of these is to shoulder the mantle of responsibility for your own life. It's natural to wish that events will sweep you along in the direction you want to go—that a corporate headhunter will call out of the blue with the perfect job, for example—but it's not a good idea to sit around waiting for "things" to happen. Nor is it particularly fruitful to dwell on how you've been crippled by your parents or any of the seemingly endless inventory of psychological dependencies—food, love, gambling, shopping, other people, what have you—being bandied about these days. "People who spend a lot of time blaming others for their problems are more likely to stay stuck in their ruts," says Penelope Russianoff, Ph.D., a New York City psychologist and faculty member at the New School for Social Research.

Second, you need to open yourself up to taking risks. We're talking not about skydiving or anything really dangerous but rather about any kind of new experience that you normally wouldn't consider trying. The operative question here is "Why not?" Taking a risk could be as simple as walking down a street you usually avoid or striking up a conversation with a stranger in the checkout line. "Whenever you make changes, you take risks. This means you confront some kind of fear, and no matter what the outcome, you gain a vitalizing sense of influence over what happens to you," says Dr. Maddi.

Finally, you need to start making changes, however small. Try to do one new thing every day. Go to work by a different route. Stand up when taking calls at your desk. Surprise your wife with concert tickets. *Anything* helps, at least to start.

We asked a number of experts for their best no-fuss tips on breaking free of ruts in several major areas of a man's life. Here's what they recommend.

WORK: GET YOUR CAREER IN GEAR

Career ruts are the most common kind. There are a number of reasons for this. We men heavily invest ourselves in our work, and we want to be challenged to test the limits of our abilities. Some jobs, however, just don't make sufficient demands on our skills and talents. At the same time, day-to-day stress is often highest at the office, so we take comfort in the routines that keep us sane. Only you can decide the proper balance. In the following tips, you should be able to find some guidance, no matter what the source of your rut.

Ask for new duties. If you always do accounts payable, ask your boss if you can do accounts receivable for two weeks. Even if the two tasks are equally routine, the change will energize you. If your boss wants to keep you where you are, ask if you can relieve him of minor responsibilities he'd rather not be bothered with, such as heading the department's recycling program. On your own, you can look for ways to streamline your unit's efficiency; some companies offer cash rewards for money-saving ideas.

Take courses. Any kind of formal learning outside the office adds excitement to your work life. But "learning" doesn't necessarily have to mean "classroom." Wilderness expeditions such as those offered by Outward Bound give participants a new take on their lives by confronting them with physical and mental challenges. Call (800) 243-8520 for information on Outward Bound.

Be a worldly traveler. Never go to another city on business without doing something fun there. What ultimately makes the trip memorable is the small jazz club you go to, the regional cuisine you eat, the historic sights you take in.

Let yourself daydream. Taking your thoughts away from work for a few minutes promotes creativity and helps you set goals for the future. "It literally changes your brain chemistry in ways that make you see things differently," says creativity consultant Ann McGee-Cooper, Ph.D., author of *You Don't Have to Go Home from Work Exhausted!*

Turn to your computer. To break out of your usual ways of approaching problems, try one of several software programs designed to promote fresh thinking. One of the best, MindLink Problem Solver, invites users to come up with ideas that are absurd or impractical and then mold them into workable strategies. Cost: around $300. Call (800) 253-1844.

Yield the chair. When reconvening conferences after a break, sit in a different chair. It changes the dynamics of the meeting and can inspire new lines of thought from weary participants.

Lean on Mr. Clean. Are you compulsively neat? Try leaving your desk messy when you go home at night. If you're naturally disorganized, tidy things up. A change in your customary level of clutter taps new reservoirs of mental power, says Dr. McGee-Cooper.

Make small changes in decor. Put a new print on your wall. Get a calendar that shows you a different picture every month rather than one that has the same drab scene or is signed "Courtesy, your friendly Allstate agent." Studies show that such small visual changes can actually make you more productive.

HOME: YOUR CASTLE OR YOUR PRISON?

Gone are the days when a man walked through his front door and was greeted by a welcoming party of a beaming wife and adoring little ones. In fact, those days probably never existed. The Ward Cleaver myth is a bust, and the reality is that coming through the front door means entering another realm where you need to work at keeping things from getting stale. "People often feel that once they're married, they don't have to worry about their life at home," says Dr. Maddi. "Five years later, they're bored to death." He and others offer the following suggestions for adding a little more interest to the humdrum details of domestic life and relationships.

Get up earlier. The world looks and feels fresher, newer and more peaceful early in the morning. Rising an hour sooner makes you feel refreshingly less time-crunched all day long. Use the extra hour to do things you usually don't, such as taking a walk or preparing the breakfast table for your wife.

Switch roles. Trade household chores with your partner. If you shop for groceries and she vacuums, swap for a week. It'll make the routine seem less dreary, and you'll each gain an appreciation of the other's responsibilities.

• •

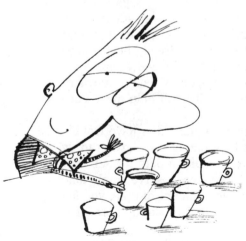

Coffee and Stress Do Mix

The stress experts have long advised us to cut back on caffeine in times of high anxiety. But now a new study suggests that coffee and stress aren't such a bad combination. For eight weeks, 21 test subjects abstained from all caffeine-containing beverages, while 43 other volunteers quaffed six cups of coffee per day. Before and after the eight-week period, researchers compared the subjects' blood pressure readings and heart rates during mental and physical stress tests. It turned out that staying off caffeine didn't make for a great improvement, and in some cases it made no difference at all. The researchers say their study calls into question the value of giving up caffeine as a means of coping with stress.

Use variety to spice meals. Mealtimes are full of entrenched routines. Instead of always eating at the kitchen table, take the food into another room. In warm weather, pack up a picnic basket and eat in a park. Break the mold of tried-and-true dishes by fixing something new or bringing dinner home from a deli.

Try a risky question. Ask your partner if she's satisfied with your relationship. Chances are that if you feel things are stagnant, she does, too. No matter what her reply, talking will build intimacy and ease estrangement.

Break destructive patterns. Identify the ways you normally respond during fights, then deliberately do something different. Say "I'm sorry" if you never do. Or if you tend to back down, don't. Point out patterns to your partner, so she tries breaking them, too.

SEX: THERE'S MORE THAN ONE WAY TO DO IT

Ho-hum sex is one of the most easily identified and quickly fixed problems two people can face, says Houston psychologist Jerome Sherman, Ph.D., past president of the American Association of Sex Educators, Counselors and Therapists. "I've seen couples who've already been to the attorney turn their relationships around by addressing long-festering sexual dissatisfaction." Hopefully, you're nowhere near that point yet. The following tips will help make sure you never are.

Give sex priority. Active couples often have trouble just being in the same place long enough for sparks to fly spontaneously. You may have to make a date for sex. But more important, when you do have sex, reserve ample time for it. "When there's only a limited amount of time, you fall into the familiar, and it can begin to feel like a chore," Dr. Sherman says.

Reminisce. Couples are more sexually daring and playful in the early days of a relationship, says Dr. McGee-Cooper. If you talk in bed about the best sex you've had and why it was good, you'll revive erotic feelings and create a sense of emotional excitement that can make a new encounter better.

Focus on foreplay. Experts say that what's usually

lacking in stale sexual relationships is a sense of intimacy, which activities such as talking, giving massages and nonintercourse sex can bolster. Try making foreplay the entire point of going to bed together.

Revise the routine. In addition to trying new positions, make love someplace other than in bed or at a different time of day than usual. Turn on lights if you usually keep them off. Quicken or slow the pace compared with your usual tempo. "There are 1,001 modifications you can make that can really set a different tone," Dr. Sherman says.

FREE TIME: DON'T BLOW IT

This is the area of life where we have the most discretion to try new things, says Dr. Simon. How we spend our free time says as much about us as our jobs. Here's what the experts suggest.

Refuse to commute. You don't *have* to leave the city after work every day. Stay in town once a month and find out what happens when the suits go home. Ask your wife or girlfriend to join you, and rent a hotel room. Go to a show or to a restaurant you've never tried in a neighborhood you don't know well.

Get off the beaten track. If you don't fish, visit a tackle shop. If you don't read novels, go browse in a bookstore. By deliberately going where you've never gone before, you may unexpectedly discover new interests.

Turn off the tube. Passive forms of entertainment such as watching TV can blacken people's moods and deepen depression, both of which make ruts worse, says Geoffrey Godbey, Ph.D., a professor of leisure studies at Pennsylvania State University.

Play with a kid. When adults play together, they often just shift the same competitive attitudes of the office to, say, the game of golf or tennis. Playing with a child taps into a purer, more imaginative sense of play that's less rule-conscious and more creative.

Get to know the other half. Make an effort to encounter people outside your profession, class, social group or race: You'll challenge your biases and gain a deeper understanding of others. One way to do it is to volunteer at a hotline service that counsels, for example, the emotionally distressed or people with AIDS. Another way is to participate in community meetings, whether about race relations or neighborhood parking. Any kind of grass-roots activism makes you feel more connected to the world around you.

Read a different newspaper. Each one has a different attitude and audience, so you'll get a slightly varied take on the day's events. If yours is a one-paper town, pick up a neighboring city's news.

Try new sports. Studies show that we gain the most enjoyment from activities we can improve in, so any sport you haven't played is a ticket out of a rut. If you're devoted to a particular competitive sport, seek out opponents who are better than you.

Work out. Exercise is good rut-breaking therapy because it produces mood-elevating brain chemicals, gives you a sense of physical control and makes you look and feel better. To keep routines from becoming monotonous, exercise with a partner whenever possible. Give workouts purpose by training

• •

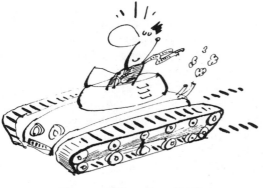

Heavy Cars Are Safer

Common wisdom holds that if you're in a small car that is struck by a large car, you'll suffer the greater injury. But size isn't everything. After analyzing thousands of fatal car collisions, engineers at General Motors concluded that it's the *weight* of the car, not the size, that matters most in how its occupants fare in crashes. For example, when a small car collided with a larger car of similar weight, the driver of the smaller car had it no worse off. So when shopping for a new car, think heavy metal.

for specific goals, such as running a 10K race. Vary your workout by altering your pace, location and scheduling.

Take mini-vacations. Instead of using all your vacation days on one big midsummer trip, spread the time across numerous long weekends. There's less pressure to guarantee yourself a good time during a short getaway than on a major vacation, says Richard Gitelson, Ph.D., also a professor of leisure studies at Pennsylvania State University. With less at stake, you're more likely to be adventurous in deciding what to do.

APPEARANCE: COLOR YOUR WORLD

Chances are you dress and groom as your job requires, and what's required for most of us is a tediously consistent business uniform of dark suit, white shirt, red tie. "Adding a touch of style can make a big difference," says Lois Fenton, author of *Dress for Excellence.* It's all in the details. Here's what she recommends.

Focus on ties. "Investing $30 in a good tie will make a whole outfit look better," Fenton says. Ties add instant flair, and snappy ties are more accepted now than they used to be.

Dress up shirts. If you always wear a button-down, try a tab collar or a straight point with a collar pin for a dressier look. "That little difference is perfect," Fenton says. "It's still very traditional, but it makes a major difference in adding polish to the whole outfit."

Invest in small touches. Minor details can lend style and class to a workaday outfit. Tuck a pocket square in the suit's breast pocket, for example (but don't wear a square that exactly matches your tie). Wear suspenders, so you look sharp even when your jacket's off. Try patterned socks (dark only) and give them exposure with low-cut loafers. Buy a classic watch or eyeglasses. And finally, Fenton suggests, get your hair cut every three weeks.

In all the advice above, there's a final lesson, a kind of rut-breaking golden rule: Let your gut instincts lead you naturally to the things that excite you and make you feel good about yourself. "Listen to what you think you want to do," Dr. Russianoff says. "Chances are it's within your grasp."

—Richard Laliberte

Don't Let This Crazy World Turn You Gray

Are you foundering in a sea of distractions? Here's how to cut through the clutter that's controlling you.

• • • • • • • • • • • • • • • • • •

SOME CALL THIS THE Age of Information. That seems an understatement. In a typical day, you're bombarded with car-phone conferences, computer mail, faxed menus from the Chinese restaurant around the corner, CNN clips, MTV hits, *USA Today* weather and sports charts, televised Senate hearings, virtual-reality games and calls from your travel agent regarding that upcoming flight to Chicago.

We should really call this the Age of Saturation, says social psychologist Kenneth Gergen, Ph.D., a professor at Swarthmore College who has studied the ways that this onslaught of information affects us. The backwash of all this change and choice, he says, is a drowning out of your sense of who you are. Instead of the comfortable assurance that deep down inside dwells the real man, you find you've become a soup of a thousand voices, images, sound bites and infographics.

A Frankenstein monster, in other words, spliced together from last night's Letterman monologue, an alluring freeze-frame from a beer ad, a phrase from a memo, a memory from a meal with a colleague in Buffalo. When you've become thoroughly saturated with powerful and seductive messages from the media, it's easy to start thinking that nothing makes sense.

Dr. Gergen describes such a state in his book *Saturated Self.* If you feel that life has been dishing out more than you can swallow, read on for Dr. Gergen's advice on how to avoid choking on it all.

Q. I'd guess there have always been busy, well-informed people, networking like mad. Why is it so much more difficult to manage life today?

A. Technology has increased enormously the number of things we can be doing, the places we can be, the people we can be with. There are tremendous advantages to that, of course. But many of us find it's all but impossible to deal with so many choices, so much information.

The first couple of hours of your day, you may have as many contacts with the world as a person once had in a full month—through the morning TV news, the paper, the people you commute and work with, plus the faxes, electronic mail and phone calls waiting for you at the office.

Q. How does this affect men in particular?

A. With increased information come increased expectations. A man 50 years ago could hold his head up simply by being sincere, reliable and hardworking. Today, he's also got to be politically savvy, knowledgeable about current events, sports and cars—not to mention physically fit, well traveled and good in bed.

Also, our role models have changed. Once upon a time we had straight shooters such as John Wayne, Humphrey Bogart and Gary Cooper to point the way. Today, we have Dustin Hoffman, Robert Redford and Paul Newman. These guys have played complex—sometimes even effeminate—roles.

Then you get Madison Avenue's image of what a man is supposed to be. Women have long had to deal with the whole concept of fashion. For men, it's a relatively new challenge: designer underwear, safari shirts, colognes, Elvis Presley *perfume*. . . . You don't know what it is anymore to be a male.

Q. How has the crush of differing roles for men affected male-female relationships?

A. The traditional marriage is one of the biggest casualties. When you have many relationships around the country with people you see only occasionally, it gets difficult to say to a particular person "Oh, you're fantastic, this must be true love." Not when you're both leaving the next day to keep up with the rest of your lives.

To say yes to one person means a thousand deaths to other fragments of your personality. The home becomes a pit stop, a place to run in and grab a sandwich.

● ●

SCREENING MESSAGES

In order to carve little time-outs into your day, "you've got to treat yourself like your top client," says Daniel L. Kegan, Ph.D., an organizational psychologist in Chicago. Decide what's important to you and do it. Stop doing things that don't make the grade. Here are some ways stress management experts suggest you can shield yourself from information overload. The key is to realize that you can't know it all and do it all, says Dr. Kegan. "Find those things that really make you feel good and give them priority."

AT WORK

- If you already read a morning paper, listen to music during your drive to work rather than a radio rehash of headlines.

- Don't get a car phone. Can't almost anything wait until you reach work?

- Avoid "in-box overload." When you get a break, sort through the pile all at once. Toss out what's not needed, pass the material to someone else, or file it for later use. Don't let papers pile up.

- Avoid the temptation to answer electronic mail messages immediately. Set aside a time period for returning messages and calls.

- Review the professional journals and newsletters you receive. Take only the most important.

● ●

Q. You suggest in your book that with all the choices, it's increasingly difficult nowadays to make decisions.

A. Right. Because you hear and see so many pros and cons for anything you might do with your life, it's easy to become frozen. Let's say you just want to sit outside and enjoy the sun. Your mind replays a news report on how sunlight ages the skin. You've also heard it's vital for success on the job to keep your youthful looks. Kind of spoils your afternoon, doesn't it? Or you want to plop down in front of the TV for a few minutes, but your on-board chorus sings out at you

• •

- Take a walk at lunchtime.
- Don't take work home every night. When you do, take only what you can realistically complete.

AT HOME

- During mealtimes, screen telephone calls with an answering machine.
- Turn off the TV set when you aren't watching something specific.
- When you are watching TV, don't channel-surf. To avoid the temptation to hop from station to station, put the remote out of reach. Check listings to decide what show you're going to watch, then stick to it. When the show is over, turn off the set.
- Take the TV sets out of your bedroom, kitchen and bathroom.
- Subscribe to one good local daily newspaper. Few people really need a community weekly, a regional and a national paper.
- Skim newspaper headlines. There's no reason to read every story.
- Make time to be alone, or with your mate, outdoors.
- Take some vacations close to home or at home.

• •

"Lazy. Couch potato." Stay late at the office, and the line is "Workaholic. Heart attack–prone."

As a result of all this information, you can become burdened with self-doubt: "Am I well traveled and well read? Am I cholesterol-conscious and trim? Am I odor-free, friendly and creative?"

Q. Where's the danger in this kind of constant self-questioning?

A. At some point you lose your sense of who you really are. You begin to feel like a fake, someone who is only pretending to be a "real professional," a "dedicated lover" or a "committed father." Actions that once seemed authentic now seem more contrived, thrown together for an audience.

Next, you begin to feel fractured. Life starts to seem preposterous and strange. You may, for instance, find yourself on the phone talking about a death in the family while in the background the kids are going wacky over some funny TV show and the neighbor is asking to borrow your lawn mower. Nothing gets digested. You get the feeling that life is

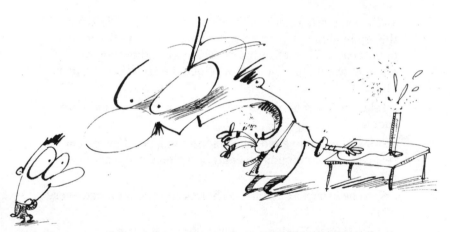

The High Price of Being Bossy

Want to do your blood pressure a favor? Stop being so bossy. Researchers found a link between social behavior and blood pressure by measuring blood pressure changes in 45 married couples during a directed discussion. In half of the discussions, the husbands were offered a shot at winning $100 if they could bring their wives around to their own point of view. Since their wives were secretly offered the same deal, the guys had their work cut out for them. (Researchers can be pretty sneaky when they want to be.) Compared with husbands who were discussing things civilly, guys trying to influence their wives had significant increases in systolic blood pressure. So next time you find yourself acting like Archie Bunker, ask yourself if it's worth sending your blood pressure skyrocketing.

a string of one damned thing after another, things that you can only witness but not really participate in.

By and by, you start to lose sight of the real you, the ability to know who you are. You lose your core.

Q. Okay, doctor, what do we do about all this? What's your prescription?

A. We need to slow down the process and put technology in a reasonable frame. All these new technologies are inviting—and advertising makes them more so. You know the kind of appeal those ads have—"Those frequent-flyer miles will earn you a free trip!" You need to remember that for every advantage, there's also a cost. To use those frequent-flyer miles, you need to spend hours planning your trip, making reservations, packing and unpacking. A better way to spend your vacation may be to simply stay home and unplug the phone.

You need periodic stoppages, times when you can really get away from it all. I suggest things such as walking in the woods, fishing, woodworking—anything that is physical or has a direct connection with the natural environment, that pulls you out of the world of symbols and language.

Q. What about marriage? Is there a role for old-fashioned monogamy in a fractured world?

A. I've found that an ongoing, traditional relationship not only is still possible but also can be a great help in coping with media saturation. I've had the remarkable good fortune of marrying someone who sees the world much as I do, and she can appreciate all my fragmentary selves, diverse impulses and role-playings. She is my safety valve, my harbor in the storm.

Q. So the anchor to sanity lies in close relationships that we preserve from the chaos of our work lives?

A. Yes, but we also need to change our points of view. We need to look for the most satisfying things in our lives—and do them. You don't *have* to see every film that's out there or every new show on TV. As you're considering an activity, ask yourself "Will doing this really make me content?"

—*Roger Yepsen*

The Most Important
Age Eraser of All

*You can turn back your biological clock 10 to 20
years in just a few months! Here's how.*

● ● ● ● ● ● ● ● ● ● ● ● ● ● ● ● ● ●

WHEN WAS THE FIRST TIME you realized you were getting
older? Was it the day you failed to beat out that grounder to
short during the company's annual softball game? Or the
time you felt out of breath after finally getting the old lawn
mower started? Or the day your new assistant confused
Simon and Garfunkel with Rocky and Bullwinkle?

Let's face it: We live in a youth culture that insists we
somehow stop aging or get out of the way. But what if you
knew of a surefire way to slow down the aging process? No,
not some miracle guacamole cream that they sell on late-
night infomercials. No, not a full-body nip and tuck.

The one proven anti-aging remedy is a lot cheaper, safer
and easier to come by. It's exercise. And many experts on
aging say it may be the next best thing to a fountain of
youth. "By taking yourself from a sedentary state to a physically trained state, you can, in effect, reduce your biological
age by 10 or 20 years," says Roy Shepard, M.D., Ph.D., a professor of applied physiology at the University of Toronto.

It is often said that exercise, if it could be bottled,
would be the most potent prescription we have for a
healthy existence. Study after study bears this out. For
example, researchers measured the effects of aging on 756
athletes, aged 35 to 94, who participated in events such as
rowing, swimming and track and field during the 1985
World Masters Games. "We found some people in their
late 60s and 70s who had about the same cardiopulmonary
fitness as you would expect from sedentary 25-year-olds,"
says Terence Kavanagh, M.D., director of the Toronto
Rehabilitation Centre. When compared with sedentary
people their own age, they averaged twice the cardiovascular fitness.

ATHLETES ARE YOUNGER

Maybe it's no surprise that amateur athletes are in better shape than the rest of us, but what is astounding is how little effort went into getting them in such good shape, says Dr. Kavanagh. Most trained less than seven hours a week in preparation for the games. "These weren't fanatical trainers in any sense," he says. "They were more typical of the average recreational sportsperson than of the elite athlete. It seems that even modest exercise can push aging back."

As a bonus, exercise can also help you live longer. In one study, 16,936 Harvard alumni, aged 35 to 74, were followed by Stanford University researchers for 12 to 16 years. Death rates were up to one-third lower among those alumni who burned more than 2,000 calories a week exercising. For an average-size man, that's equivalent to running or walking three miles a day.

And just because you stopped exercising when you left college doesn't mean that you can't get a lease on longer life. The Stanford researchers concluded that people who start exercising between the ages of 35 and 55 can probably add two years to their life expectancy. Even if you start exercising in your 70s, you can add an extra six months to your life.

A HEALTHY MIX

If you mix exercise with other healthful practices, your prospects for a longer life become even greater, says Kenneth Manton, Ph.D., assistant director of Duke University's Center for Demographic Studies. In addition to exercising, you should stay slim, not smoke, keep your cholesterol low and follow a low-fat diet, says Dr. Manton.

He came to this conclusion after using an innovative computer program to reanalyze data from several major population studies, including the famed 20-year Framingham Heart Study. He concluded that a healthful lifestyle including regular exercise, begun at age 30, has the potential to extend the average life expectancy in the United States by as much as 15 years.

But it's exercise itself that many doctors believe will help make *all* your years—no matter how many there are—productive and disease-free.

Consider what can happen to the body when it *stops* exercising. A Swedish physiologist asked five young men to remain bedridden 24 hours a day for three weeks to study their bodies' physiological responses. All the men experienced a drop in their aerobic capacity equivalent to almost 20 years of aging!

"A lot of the effects of aging are self-inflicted," Dr. Kavanagh says. "The less you do, the easier you fatigue. And the more you fatigue, the less you are able to do."

Breaking that cycle is critical. "I think it's just common sense," Dr. Kavanagh says. "Just look around you, and you'll see that the people who are physically active work harder, tire less and enjoy themselves a lot more.

"Regular physical activity is excellent for everyone," Dr. Kavanagh says. "But it has to be regular; it can't be inconsis-

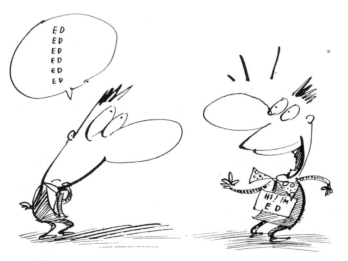

What You Say
Is What You Get

Researchers at Washington University School of Medicine in St. Louis say your short-term memory works best when you silently repeat words rather than visualizing them in your mind's eye. In a study, people who used speech-based mental processing recalled more information than those who relied on visual imagery.

tent. It needs to be something that you do at least three times a week."

HUFF AND PUFF

Which brings us to the question: What kind of exercise is best to hold back the aging process? First, anything aerobic. Huff-and-puff exercise, such as swimming, running and cycling, is the most powerful weapon against many of the effects of aging, according to the numerous studies.

Aerobic workouts are important because without adequate oxygen, the body doesn't perform at its best, Dr. Kavanagh says.

"If you let yourself go to pot, you're artificially reducing your oxygen uptake. If you do that, you really can't function well. You think slower, you move slower. You're just less capable of taking advantage of this world," he says.

So how do you take advantage of this high-octane energy booster? What do you do if you've already slumped into a sedentary lifestyle?

Start slowly. You don't have to get off the couch and launch into a five-mile run on your first day. Brisk walking is an excellent aerobic exercise for beginners, doctors say, because it is easy and can give you all the health-enhancing and age-resisting benefits of more strenuous aerobic activities, such as jogging. Walking will also get you in condition for more rigorous activities such as biking and swimming.

Aerobic exercise is just one component of an anti-aging package. You should also consider some form of weight training, experts say. Researchers at Tufts University found that weight training significantly improved the muscle strength of 12 previously sedentary men, aged 60 to 72. During the three months of weight lifting, muscle strength increases ranged from 107 percent to 226 percent, and total muscle mass increased by an average of 10 percent. These gains were similar to those reported by healthy younger men undergoing a comparable training regimen.

The bottom line: Activity beats aging. Working out not only will help you feel younger, it will make you look younger, too.

—Doug Dollemore

Part 2

HEALTHY EATS

Men and the Vitamins That Love Them

Your doctor is probably taking vitamins, and for some pretty good reasons, too. So why aren't you?

• • • • • • • • • • • • • • • • • •

IF YOU'RE LIKE MOST MEN, you probably haven't taken vitamin pills since your mother doled out those little ones shaped like Fred and Wilma Flintstone. In those days it seemed to make sense, because you ate primarily jelly sandwiches and orange Popsicles, and besides, your mother stood there and watched until you swallowed your vitamin. As an adult who eats fruits and vegetables regularly (okay, at least once in a while), I figured I was getting all the vitamins

I needed from my diet. At least that's what I figured until I started reading some of the latest scientific studies on vitamins. Now I take my vitamins every day, even when my mother's not visiting.

It started with a couple of big conferences where the nation's top nutrition researchers presented, in as dry a manner as possible, some astounding new findings. The Cliffs Notes summary is that vitamins are now recognized to play a role in the health and vigor of every organ in the body, from skin and bones to the nervous and immune systems, right up to and including the brain. Studies show that being well supplied in vitamins can lower your cholesterol, help make wounds heal faster, raise your sperm count and make you more resistant to colds and flu, asthma, cataracts—even gum disease.

MORE TO THE PICTURE

But that's not all. Certain powerhouse vitamins, particularly C, E and beta-carotene, may also have a protective benefit against the effects of aging and some diseases. When administered in high doses, all three have been shown to strengthen the body's resistance to certain cancers. The evidence is particularly strong for cancers of the stomach, esophagus, pancreas, mouth and lungs. Vitamins C and E and beta-carotene may also protect against heart attack by keeping cholesterol from turning into artery-clogging sludge. Some researchers now believe that having a high intake of these vitamins may prove to be as important to heart health as lowering dietary fat. There's also evidence that beta-carotene boosts immune functions in AIDS patients.

These reports are changing the way even the usually staid members of the scientific community look at supplements. "We used to think of vitamins strictly in terms of what you needed to prevent short-term deficiencies," says Simin N. Meydani, D.V.M., Ph.D., chief of the nutritional immunology laboratory at the U.S. Department of Agriculture (USDA) Human Nutrition Research Center on Aging at Tufts University. "Now we're starting to think about what the optimal level of vitamins is for lifelong health and to prevent age-associated diseases."

The question this originally raised for me is: Do I need

to take pills to get vitamins at these "optimal" levels? As I said, I'd always felt my eating was pretty good, but with this question in mind, I decided to put my diet to the test. I recorded what I ate on a recent rainy Saturday when I had nothing better to do than think of what I was eating. Then I had the nutritional content analyzed. I must confess that what follows is better than my usual fare, but please bear with me. I'm trying to make a point here.

Breakfast
1 bowl oatmeal with skim milk
1 banana
1 glass apple juice
1 bagel with jam

Lunch
1 turkey sandwich on whole wheat, with lettuce and tomato
2 large pretzels
1 peach
2 fig bars
1 glass iced tea

Midafternoon snack
1 apple
2 nacho cheese rice cakes

Dinner
1 tossed salad, made with iceberg lettuce, chick-peas, onion
  and tomato and topped with nonfat blue cheese dressing
1 baked chicken breast
1 cup brown rice
1 cup steamed fresh zucchini
1 beer

Late-night snack
2 cups air-popped popcorn

I've got to hand it to me. That was an exemplary diet—at least for that one day. It was low in fat and high in fiber

(continued on page 28)

- -

GET WHAT YOU NEED

If you've ever been to the vitamin section of your local drugstore, you know what a bewildering array of choices there is—everything from colorful kiddie pills to obscure amino acids with five-syllable names. Here's a map to help you through the maze.

THE BASICS

■ **Multivitamin/mineral supplement**

Benefit: Taking a supplement that provides 100 percent of the Recommended Dietary Allowances (RDAs) for all the basic vitamins will ensure that you're getting at least adequate levels of these nutrients even if they're not in your diet. A good supplement should include beta-carotene (or vitamin A), the B vitamins (thiamine, riboflavin, niacin, biotin, pantothenic acid, folate, B_6 and B_{12}) as well as vitamins C, D, E and K.

Many formulas also include minerals in ranges of 50 to 100 percent of the RDAs. Be sure yours has at least 100 percent of the RDAs for potassium, magnesium, selenium and zinc and at least 100 micrograms of chromium. These five are the minerals men need most.

THE EXTRAS

Some individual vitamins are worth taking in amounts several times higher than their RDAs. To do that, do not take added multivitamins. Most of the nutrients in a multivitamin aren't needed in amounts much beyond the RDAs; others aren't good for you in high doses. Instead, add the supplements below. For safety, the *total* amount of nutrients you get from your multivitamin and additional supplements should not exceed the levels recommended.

■ **Vitamin C**

RDA: 60 milligrams

Recommended supplement: 250 to 1000 milligrams

(continued)

- -

● ●

GET WHAT YOU NEED—*CONTINUED*

Possible benefits: Boosts the immune system to ward off colds and other illnesses; guards against cancer, heart disease and stroke; keeps gums and teeth healthy; prevents cataracts; speeds wound healing; counteracts asthma; prevents infertility by maintaining sperm quality.

Good dietary sources: Orange juice, red peppers, strawberries, grapefruit juice, broccoli and papaya.

■ Vitamin E

RDA: 14 international units

Recommended supplement: 100 to 400 international units

Possible benefits: Prevents buildup of artery-clogging plaque; boosts the immune system; protects against stroke and cancer; prevents cataracts.

Good dietary sources: Almonds, wheat germ, peanuts, pecans and canola oil.

■ Beta-carotene

RDA: None established, but 6 milligrams would give the equivalent of the RDA for vitamin A

Recommended supplement: 15 to 30 milligrams

Possible benefits: Boosts the immune system; protects against cancer, heart disease and stroke; maintains good vision; keeps skin healthy.

Good dietary sources: Carrots, pumpkin, sweet potatoes, spinach and cantaloupe.

■ Chromium

RDA: None established

Recommended supplement: 50 to 200 micrograms

● ●

Possible benefits: Lowers cholesterol; stimulates muscle growth; controls blood sugar.

Good dietary sources: Wheat germ, American cheese, dried prunes and chromium-fortified brewer's yeast tablets.

■ Selenium

RDA: 70 micrograms

Recommended supplement: 70 to 200 micrograms

Possible benefits: Boosts the immune system; protects against heart disease, stroke and cancers of the colon, rectum and lungs.

Good dietary sources: Shrimp, lobster, brewer's yeast, whole-grain cereals and breads.

Safety: Toxic in high doses. Do not exceed 200 micrograms.

Experts recommend that when shopping for supplements, you avoid spending extra money on frills. Terms such as *chelated, enhanced bioavailability* and *natural* aren't meaningful except as marketing ploys.

Also, check the expiration date on the label. To guarantee freshness, that date should be at least two years in the future.

It's best to buy brand-name vitamins such as those bearing the label of a drugstore chain. Because the Food and Drug Administration regulates vitamins as foods, not drugs, quality can vary. Most brand-name vitamins are made by large, reliable companies.

and included a nice variety of fruits and vegetables. But here's what I discovered: My day's food barely covered me for the government's Recommended Dietary Allowances (RDAs) for most vitamins and was below par in a few, notably vitamins C and E and beta-carotene. Okay, I could have gotten more vitamin C by drinking orange juice instead of apple juice, and I could have gotten more beta-carotene by eating a few carrots or some broccoli. Adding vitamin E is a little trickier, since it's concentrated in foods I try to avoid, such as cooking oils and full-fat salad dressings, and foods I seldom eat, such as sunflower seeds, almonds and pecans.

ON THE SAFE SIDE

Taking a vitamin pill just to be on the safe side didn't seem like such a bad idea. A lot of experts agree. "Taking supplements is a practical way for a man to make sure he's getting all the vitamins and minerals he needs," says Jeffrey Blumberg, Ph.D., associate director of the USDA Human Nutrition Research Center on Aging.

This advice goes double for most men, since on average only 9 percent of us consume three or more vegetables and two or more fruits daily, as recommended by the government. "A lot of men are just barely getting by," says John Erdman, Jr., Ph.D., director of the division of nutritional sciences at the University of Illinois. "They may get more colds or take longer to recover from setbacks to their health."

For a basic daily supplement, you want a pill that contains 100 percent of the RDA for all the vitamins. Also, check the label to be sure that the blend includes 100 percent of the RDA for potassium, magnesium, selenium and zinc, which are minerals men need more than women. Chromium, another important mineral for men, has no established RDA. Be sure the formula includes at least 100 micrograms of chromium. Don't worry if the supplement is low in iron. Most men get more than enough of that from their diets.

BEYOND THE RDA

The next point underscored by the new research is whether even a multivitamin is sufficient for optimum health.

In all the studies where specific vitamins provided protection against cancer and heart disease, they were taken in doses several times higher than the RDA. Going above the RDA isn't supported by government advice, but some researchers think it's a good idea. "The potential benefits appear significant, and the risks are very small—including cost, which is pennies a day," says Dr. Blumberg.

The vitamins in question, C, E and beta-carotene, are all antioxidants, compounds that attack toxic particles called free radicals. Free radicals are damaging oxygen molecules produced naturally in thousands of chemical reactions each day. They're what makes steak left on your kitchen counter turn brown; they're what makes metal rust. In your body, they cause skin to toughen and wrinkle and blood vessels to lose flexibility, and they also weaken the immune system, making you more prone to cancer and other diseases.

Antioxidant supplements would seem to be an especially good idea for city dwellers who are exposed to a lot of air pollution: Hidden in the plumes of smoke belching out of factories are tons of free radicals. Cigarette smoking also produces free radicals; some research suggests that smokers who quit may return to normal health faster if they take extra supplements of vitamins C and E and beta-carotene.

Nobody's yet sure what the optimal dosages are for the antioxidants. But Dr. Blumberg offers the following safe ranges in which you might expect to gain a disease-fighting benefit.

■ Vitamin C: 250 to 1000 milligrams daily (RDA: 60 milligrams)

■ Vitamin E: 100 to 400 international units daily (RDA: 14 international units)

■ Beta-carotene: 15 to 30 milligrams daily (RDA: none established)

These numbers are all 3 to 28 times the recommended minimum amounts, but since none of these vitamins is dangerous at such levels, they won't harm you. If you want to get high doses of antioxidants, you'll have to take supplements, since it would be extremely difficult to get this much from foods. For example, you'd have to eat about 13 oranges to get 1000 milligrams of vitamin C.

You can buy antioxidant nutrients individually at your drugstore. Even easier, you can get high but safe levels of vitamins C and E and beta-carotene blended in specially marked multivitamin formulas. Look for "antioxidant-rich" or words to that effect on the label.

If you're wondering why your doctor hasn't told you about any of this, the reason most often given by health-care types is not that they oppose supplements but that they're afraid you might abandon all attempts to eat well and just pop a vitamin every day. I think you're a lot more intelligent than that. So don't ask your doctor whether you should take vitamins; ask him if *he* does. "Every person I know in the nutrition research field is taking supplements," says Bruce Ames, Ph.D., director of the National Institute of Environmental Health Sciences at the University of California, Berkeley.

• •

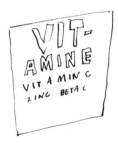

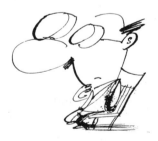

Vitamins in Sight

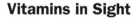

Taking antioxidant vitamins (C, E and beta-carotene) and the mineral zinc may prevent macular degeneration. This age-related eye disease causes eyesight to deteriorate in 5 percent of the population over age 45. In a small pilot study, between 30 and 35 percent of patients with macular degeneration showed improvement after taking vitamin and mineral supplements. According to ophthalmologist David Newsome, M.D., nearly one-third of Americans with the disease do not receive the U.S. Recommended Daily Allowances of antioxidant vitamins. Megadoses of certain vitamins can be harmful.

BE A SKEPTIC

Even those who endorse vitamin supplementation will advise you to maintain a skeptical attitude about the more nebulous claims for vitamins that are less well established by research. There's little evidence, for example, that the vitamins in foods or supplements can increase your brain power, cure baldness—or put you in touch with Shirley MacLaine's ancestors.

That's okay with me. The *documented* claims for taking a daily vitamin are powerful enough. "You still need to concentrate on eating right," says Dr. Blumberg. "But you can look at supplements as a low-cost form of health insurance."

—Richard Allan

Eat Like a Man

How even a bachelor can get decent nutrition without having to actually enter a kitchen.

• • • • • • • • • • • • • • • • • •

NOTHING, THEY SAY, changes a man like marriage. What is a good, useful telltale signal of marriage's impact? Try food. You can tell the difference right away between a married man and a bachelor by the questions each asks about food. For example, a married man is likely to ask something like this: "Hey, honey, what's for dinner?" A bachelor question goes something like this: "Why is it we can put a man on the moon but we can't solve the twin dilemmas of diet and laundry by making an edible gym sock that, when lightly microwaved, tastes like pizza?"

Every bachelor has a unique tale of heartbreak and anguish, of loneliness and despair, of cheap pickup lines and memorable nights with beauty queens. But all bachelors have one thing in common: They all gotta eat.

The bad news is, sometimes you gotta eat alone. The

good news is, you can live like a bachelor and still eat like a man—provided you're willing to pick up a few general principles and apply them to single-guy eats.

Statistics say single guys croak early, while married men live long and prosper. Food probably has something to do with that. The marital board is lush and regular and usually has something green on it. In a bachelor fridge, only the cheese is green. You could die eating bachelor grub. So here, as an appetizer, are five simple rules for surviving the nutritional potholes on the solitary road, followed by a bite-by-bite exploration of the principal bachelor food groups.

These may at first seem elementary, Watson, but if you're like most bachelors, you haven't been paying much attention to them anyway, so they bear repeating.

1. Mom's Law. For most of us, women have been the Kitchen Kops, working the dietary beat since Day One. For example, there's the Universal Principle of the Golden Nutritional Mean, also known as Mom's Law. Mom's Law says: Eat three squares a day. No way? No time? Then graze. Eat small portions several times a day. Mom probably once told you this was a bad idea, but she's changed her mind. Now it's okay, as long as you make your snacks something remotely healthy: a piece of fruit, a bagel, air-popped popcorn or a bag of pretzels. The idea here is to never go without eating for longer than five hours. Brain drain and fatigue lie that way.

Mom's Law also has a predictable corollary: Don't skip breakfast. Eat a slice of toast with a glass of fruit juice, a bowl of cereal or three of any fast-food chain's pancakes. (The syrup's okay, but skip the butter.) Something in the morning jump-starts the system and helps you manage your eating throughout the day.

2. Svelteness by the numbers. For every 3,500 calories you eat beyond what your body burns, you'll gain a pound. For every 3,500-calorie deficit, you'll lose a pound. For instance, the rough requirement for most average-size men is 2,500 calories a day. Let's say you're an average guy, and let's say part of your daily diet is two Kit Kat bars. That's 460 calories a day of Kit Kat nutrition. Skip those bars, and you're down to around 2,000 calories a day. If you suck up only 2,000 calories every day, you'll lose about a pound a week on average. Exercise is excellent, of course, and helps your body burn up, rather than store, calories. But exercise alone won't do it. You must reduce your calorie intake, too.

3. The Iron Law of Fat. Avoid it when you can. There. Read the package label or the handouts many restaurants provide. Normally, the amount of fat is given in grams per serving. Each gram of fat provides 9 calories. Multiply the number of grams of fat by 9. Divide that number by the total number of calories in a serving. What you get is the percentage of calories from fat. Think hard about anything that gets 30 percent or more of its total calories from fat. For example, four frozen fish sticks have 12 grams of fat and 280 calories, which may not look too bad. But $12 \times 9 \div 280$ reveals that 39 percent of the calories come from fat. Bad.

If this is too much mathematics for you, think of it this way: Try to keep it under three grams of fat per 100 calories.

4. The Equally Iron Law of Salt. Don't add salt to anything. Food preparers habitually oversalt. The National Academy of Sciences suggests no more than 2400 milligrams of sodium a day, or about a teaspoon of salt. Remember that number: 2400. Look at the food labels. Some frozen chicken entrées, for example, contain up to 1000 milligrams, and some frozen chicken complete dinners exceed 2000. That's a pillar of salt in anybody's book, especially when you consider salt's link to life-shortening high blood pressure.

5. The cholesterol controversy. A little while ago, bad-boy foods such as whole eggs, which contain bucknaked cholesterol, were seen as heart stoppers. Eat an egg and die, the science boys said.

They were sort of right: It's a good idea to eat less rather than more. But the new rule says not to eliminate cholesterol completely unless there's a medical reason to do so. The most recent recommendation is to top out at about 300 milligrams of cholesterol a day. A fast-food scrambled egg platter can give you that or more; you wouldn't want to do too many of those.

That's all the law you need. Now for some science.

Nutritionists love charts showing the basic food groups,

with nice little illustrations in case you've forgotten what a leafy vegetable looks like. You should eat a little from the dairy group, lots from the fruits and vegetables, a little less meat and a little more fish and chicken and lots more things like beans.

But we know that for single men, real life isn't so neat. To the extent that a busy man thinks at all about nutrition's little laws, he probably sees the world of chow organized around the BFGs, or *bachelor food groups*.

THE DRIVE-THRU FOOD GROUP

This group includes everything you get from chains, roach coaches, vending machines and lots of restaurants, including the cafeteria at work.

If you're a man on the move, you're at a disadvantage diet-wise, and food preparers can shovel just about anything they want into you. But enough of you have spoken up that chains and restaurants are now calling attention to low-fat or low-calorie specials and vegetarian offerings. Not all are as lean as they would have you believe. But check these items out.

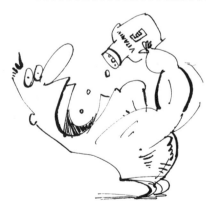

Give Yourself E
for Painless Effort

After a raging session of weight lifting, you feel like Superman—until the next morning, when you shuffle around stiffly like an old geezer. A study at the U.S. Department of Agriculture Human Nutrition Research Center on Aging at Tufts University suggests that taking vitamin E before a workout may keep you from getting so sore. Apparently, it works by limiting the damage to your muscle tissue that occurs when oxygen streams through it—a result of all that exercise. Vitamin E also appears to help reduce swelling, which contributes to soreness.

■ A Carl's Jr. Lite Potato gets only 3 percent of its calories from fat and contains no cholesterol and a mere 60 milligrams of sodium.

■ A McDonald's McLean Deluxe sandwich gets 28 percent of its calories from fat and delivers slightly more than 650 milligrams of sodium.

■ Hardee's grilled chicken breast sandwich gets 26 percent of its calories from fat and contains acceptable levels of sodium and cholesterol. In general, chicken sandwiches are healthy, provided they aren't made from big slabs of fried chicken.

■ Long John Silver's baked fish with lemon crumbs gets a scant 17 percent of its calories from fat and has 680 milligrams of sodium.

■ El Pollo Loco's flame-broiled chicken salad gets 16 percent of its calories from fat and contains only 375 milligrams of sodium.

In fact, salads, generally, are a good idea. You knew that. But the only way to keep them good, friend, is to keep your paws away from the dressings. Exceptions: a drop or two of oil with all the vinegar you want; any of the Kraft Free dressings, which have no fat at all; any other low-fat dressings that get less than 30 percent of their calories from fat.

Meanwhile, avoid these.

■ Breakfast sausage platters: just about anyone's. You're looking at 60 percent fat and 1000 milligrams of sodium, minimum.

■ Tricky salads: Chef and taco salads can get 40 to 60 percent of their calories from fat. And sodium for both can top 1000 milligrams.

■ Tricky sandwiches: Croissant sandwiches with egg and bacon or cheese get 60 percent or more of their calories from fat.

■ Burgers: Sorry, but the truth is, McDonald's is about the only place with a burger that gets less than 30 percent of its calories from fat. And almost everything burgerlike contains from one-third to one-half of all the salt you should be consuming in an entire day—and that's before you start salting it.

• •

THE SINGLE MAN'S FOOD GROUPS AT A GLANCE

The Drive-Thru Food Group. If you're a man on the move, you're at a disadvantage, diet-wise. Salad and grilled chicken are the healthiest choices.

The Food That Drives to You Group. If it's pizza, hold the pepperoni. If it's Chinese, head toward the chicken end of the menu.

The Supermarket Food Group. The frozen-food department at the supermarket is the singles bar of the microwaving singles set. Read the fine print before you buy.

The Do-It-Yourself Food Group. Stuff you buy and actually cook for yourself. In other words, spaghetti. Watch the meatballs.

The Danger Food Group. Things you want go easy on. Occasional forays into the land of alcohol and fat won't destroy you. Wrecking a man's body takes time.

• •

■ Deep-fried fish: It's likely to be fattier than a burger.

Sometimes the adjectives are a giveaway: Stay away from anything described as "creamed" or "creamy," "au gratin" or "buttery." There are alternatives, fortunately. Look for these words: "grilled," "charbroiled," "flame-broiled," "baked," "roasted," "boiled," "in its own sauce/juice."

THE FOOD THAT DRIVES TO YOU GROUP

Pizza. What sort of shameless food would come knocking at your front door? If you're having it brought in, it's probably pizza. Pizza's not necessarily awful food, but it's hardly perfect either. A pizza secret: Simpler is better. Cut down on the cheese. If you can hold the pepperoni, do so. Vegetables are fine.

A slice of basic cheese pizza gets 28 percent of its calories from fat and contains about 700 milligrams of sodium. Not bad, right? But the same pizza with extra cheese and pepperoni can double the fat and push sodium over 1000 milligrams. That's about how it runs across the big pizza board.

Chicken. Avoid fried chicken. Period.

Wok on wheels. One of the hipper trends in home delivery is Asian food, mostly Chinese and Thai. Many of these dishes are high in oil and sodium. To cut down on both, always get steamed rice instead of fried. Avoid egg rolls, fried dumplings and higher-fat dishes such as those using pork, and head toward the chicken end of the menu. Or better yet, choose from the vegetable list—get it steamed.

THE SUPERMARKET FOOD GROUP

The supermarket food group is composed of two classes: (1) food you buy to eat, and (2) food you feel you have to buy when you're really just there to meet women. The frozen-food department at the supermarket is the singles bar of the microwaving singles set. Since you have to buy something to provide decent cover, you need to heed the rules of smart shopping. In general:

■ Again, simpler is better. For example, frozen chicken pot pies are almost always higher in everything you don't want than roasted chicken entrées.

■ Read the fine print. Even if an item is low in, say, calories, it might be a killer when it comes to sodium or fat. Also, don't get caught believing that "lower-fat" is synonymous with "low-fat." "Lower" just means it has less than it used to, which may have been a hell of a lot.

■ Cups of noodles may have only 200 to 300 calories but can top 40 percent of calories from fat and are loaded with salt.

■ Some brands of "light" batter-dipped fish get more than half of their calories from fat, which is actually more than some regular fish fillets or fish sticks.

■ Vienna sausages are out of the question. The tiny weenies are above 80 percent of calories from fat and run as high as 750 milligrams of sodium per serving.

It's not entirely hopeless. There are a number of frozen dishes that will do when the microwave is all you have time for. All the entrées and dinners below meet our low-fat standard. Just be sure to fit their sodium contribution into what you're getting the rest of the day.

■ Healthy Choice roasted turkey and mushrooms in gravy gets 14 percent of its 200 calories from fat and has 380 milligrams of sodium.

■ Weight Watchers shrimp marinara with linguini has only 150 calories and less than a gram of fat. Sodium: 390 milligrams.

■ Le Menu Healthy golden glazed chicken gets only 8 percent of its 330 calories from fat and has 420 milligrams of sodium.

■ Budget Gourmet Light and Healthy teriyaki beef has 270 calories, 6 grams of fat and 520 milligrams of sodium.

■ Stouffer's Lean Cuisine three-cheese French bread pizza gets 27 percent of its 330 calories from fat and has 350 milligrams of sodium.

THE DO-IT-YOURSELF FOOD GROUP

The DIY food group includes the stuff you buy and actually cook for yourself. So we're talking spaghetti here, right? Right. Spaghetti contains almost no fat and won't salt your innards for you. Tomato spaghetti sauce is ambrosia for the health-conscious bachelor. But if you want to get downright Italo-cool, simply heat ½ teaspoon of olive oil and mix in any or all of these: a clove of minced garlic, a handful of sunflower seeds, some chopped parsley, a sliced Japanese eggplant or Italian squash, some sun-dried tomatoes, red pepper flakes or capers. Toss with pasta, and you've got a fine meal.

See, single guys need style in the kitchen as much as elsewhere, and nothing makes you feel more like the master of your own destiny than going out to the supermarket, stalking some real food, bagging it at the checkout and bringing it back to the "bach-cave" for a little prep.

For instance, buy some boneless chicken breasts. Because they're also skinless, nearly all the fat has been pulled off for you. Put the breasts in a pan with some low-sodium canned chicken stock and a few slices of garlic. Cover and simmer until the chicken's done. Zap, a meal.

THE DANGER FOOD GROUP

Supermarket roulette: Most types of coleslaw, hot dogs and sausages such as pepperoni, chorizo and liverwurst are sky-high in fat, while soufflés, whole eggs, ice cream, custard and even shrimp are disproportionately high in cholesterol.

The vile and dreaded salt monsters come cleverly disguised as dill pickles, canned soups, specialty items such as onion or garlic salt, soy sauce, cheese, salted nuts, olives and barbecue and curry sauces, not to mention innocent-seeming cottage cheese. Some lunch meats are more than 50 percent fat and contain 2000 milligrams of sodium per serving. Stick to chicken, turkey and seafoods such as water-packed tuna. Just be sure to hold the mayo and the Russian dressing.

Alcohol, the liquid idiot, is high in calories and has practically nothing else of any value except the ability to make you forget your own true love and the nation's deficit. But you knew that already, didn't you?

That's the nutrition part. But are we not men? Death will not follow instantaneously upon ingestion of moderate quantities of any of the above; nor will occasional bacheloresque forays into nutritional vice wreck your constitution or immediately balloon you into obesity. Destroying a man's body takes time. Which also means that with a little effort, and sense, you can maintain your peace of mind and body weight and help yourself avoid bodily malfunction.

Even if you're a bachelor.

—Bruce Henstell

Power Nutrition

Adopt this power eating plan,
and all-day energy will be yours.

• • • • • • • • • • • • • • • • •

YOUR COMPANY CERTAINLY EXPECTS a lot for those jumbo bucks it pays you. Sixty-hour weeks, business trips on weekends, decision-intensive, nerve-splintering workdays. You need plenty of mental and physical stamina to get through it all. A proper diet can help. The problem is time. Who has enough to keep up with all the latest nutritional advice, gather the necessary ingredients of a healthy eating regimen and carefully ingest said ingredients at the right moment and in the correct amounts? When it comes to nutrition, what you want are the fast facts: "What do I need to eat so that I can function at maximum efficiency? How can I eat it in a way that will waste the least amount of time?"

To the busy man, the concept of three nutritious meals a day is little more than a fairy tale. Unpredictable working hours, surprise business lunches and deadlines that should have been met yesterday all conspire to keep you from maintaining anything close to the eating schedule your body and mind require to operate like a lean, mean living machine. But even if you do manage to get in those three squares, you could be falling short.

EAT FOUR OR FIVE MEALS

"One of the most important stamina rules is that your body needs its fuel in moderate doses throughout the day to keep energy nutrients optimally available at the cellular level," says Peter M. Miller, Ph.D., executive director of the Hilton Head Health Institute and author of *The Hilton Head Executive Stamina Program.* "I actually counsel people to eat between four and five times a day."

At first you might think that following this advice would make you a fat man rather than an energized one. But if we use an analogy Dr. Miller is fond of, the logic becomes a bit more apparent. Think about your car. Do you fill it up only after it runs out of gas? Or do you quite sensibly top off the tank at regular intervals, making sure that you always have enough fuel to go the distance?

"Many executives will grab a cup of coffee and a Danish around 8:00 A.M. and then put off lunch until 2:00 in the afternoon. Meanwhile, they run out of gas by midday and spend a couple of hours operating at well below their peak stamina level," notes Dr. Miller. "By eating four to five times a day, you avoid running low."

This isn't meant to give you license to stuff yourself regularly. After all, you don't try to cram ten gallons of gas into your car when you need only five to fill the tank. "What I am suggesting is that you reduce the amount of food you eat at any one time, so you can spread the same amount of calories more evenly over the day," says Dr. Miller.

Eating less, but more frequently, makes good sense for another reason. "The larger the meal, the more time it takes to digest," says Dr. Miller. "And the process of digestion requires increased blood and oxygen flow to the stomach and intestines. This represents energy that will not be available for the brain and muscles to use." In other words, the bigger the meal, the more time you'll spend operating in that groggy, after-the-Thanksgiving-feast state of mind. It's not where you want to be when you have important decisions to make after lunch.

USE HIGH-OCTANE FOOD

While your fueling schedule is an important component of your stamina level, the kind of fuel you use also makes a difference. A high-octane diet is one that is high in complex carbohydrates, such as those found in whole grains and vegetables. "To ensure that you are receiving the large amounts of glucose that your body needs to maintain maximum energy, your basic fuel mix should be 60 percent carbohydrates, 15 percent protein and no more than 25 percent fat daily," says Dr. Miller. "Many people subscribe to the old belief that protein is where you get your energy, but this is not exactly true. Depend on foods such as vegetables, cereals, pasta, bread, potatoes and fruits to give you the carbohydrates your body needs to manufacture a steady supply of glucose. Rather than having a steak and fries for lunch, for example, you would do much better ordering a fruit platter, salad or perhaps pasta primavera. Fewer calories, more carbohydrates is the rule."

Midmorning or late afternoon (assuming you eat break-

● ●

Take This to Breakfast, Lunch and Dinner

You'll get more from your beta-carotene vitamin supplements if you take them at mealtimes. In a recent study, people who took 51 milligrams of beta-carotene divided over three meals absorbed three times as much of the vitamin as people who took one 51-milligram dose at breakfast.

fast at 7:00 A.M. and lunch at 1:00 P.M. or 2:00 P.M.) is when you want to go for the additional mini-meal or snack. Dr. Miller suggests any of the following for a perfect pickup when your glucose levels are sagging.

1 medium banana
1 orange
¼ cup raisins
5 dates
¼ honeydew melon
½ medium cantaloupe
3 medium apricots
½ medium apple
2 figs

To counteract dehydration, be sure to drink fluids throughout the day. "One of the things we know about energy is that when your body loses fluid, you tend to get tired," says Dr. Miller. "Executives should take particular care, since they frequently become dehydrated due to stuffy work environments as well as time spent in airplanes."

WATCH THE CAFFEINE

But you do want to go easy on coffee, colas and other caffeine-laden beverages. "Since caffeine is a diuretic, those drinks will only aggravate the problem," says Dr. Miller. He suggests a "stamina spritzer": 60 percent orange juice and 40 percent carbonated water, served very cold. It also makes a good drink to help get you started in the morning, he says.

In the quest for stamina, many a man may wonder if some additional vitamins are in order. "My feeling," says Dr. Miller, "is that a well-rounded diet is the most important source of nutrients. But if you feel that you're guilty of some rather patchy eating habits, you may need to take a multivitamin with a mineral supplement for nutritional insurance."

In short, Miller's eating program for busy men is this: small, nutrition-packed meals, plenty of healthy snacks, a preponderance of complex carbohydrates, increased fluid intake and a multivitamin/mineral supplement if necessary.

—*Mark Golin*

Male Myths of Weight Loss

*Dropping a few pounds will be a snap once
you discard these common misconceptions.*

••••••••••••••••••

ON THE SUBJECT OF WEIGHT LOSS, misconceptions
abound. Women, for example, think that we men don't care
about our weight. Any one of us can confirm that this is not
true. It's just that we don't obsess about our weight and we
don't go on diets as often as women. We're rightfully skeptical about food fads. We go to bookstores for Tom Clancy
techno-thrillers, not 30-day recipe books. We believe weight
loss, like a military operation, is something that should be
undertaken only when truly necessary. We'll cut our flab a
little slack, but when things really get out of line, we're ready
to take action.

The question is how to lose the extra pounds with the
least amount of bother and fuss.

As fad-wary men, we tend to rely on time-honored
strategies for dropping pounds. Recently, however, there's
been a lot of new thinking based on solid research about
proper food choices and exercise, the two key elements of
any weight loss plan. Think of it as new intelligence in the
weight loss war. If you're using old information, you'll probably end up working harder than necessary to lose those
pounds. Efficiency—now that's something most of us can
sink our teeth into.

We asked a panel of experts to point out how commonly
held beliefs have changed. What follows is a list of eight
weight loss myths that often influence men and the truths
that have replaced them. Changing these old ways of thinking, our experts say, will make it considerably easier to get
rid of that excess baggage.

1. Starches make you fat. Not so. Stick-to-the-ribs
fare such as potatoes, breads and pasta is the fastest-burning
food you can eat. All are carbohydrates, which provide the
body's main source of ready-to-use fuel. Experts recommend
that the greatest share of our diet—60 percent—be com-

posed of this high-octane nutrient. "Only a tiny percentage of carbohydrates is ever converted to fat in the body," says Adam Drewnowski, Ph.D., director of the human nutrition program at the University of Michigan's School of Public Health.

Still, misconceptions linger on this score because of studies suggesting that overweight people crave starchy food, which implies that carbohydrates foster obesity. Dr. Drewnowski has found otherwise in studies showing that what people really crave is fat, which turns to flab far more easily than either carbohydrates or protein.

It's easy to confuse high-carbohydrate foods with high-fat ones because the two ingredients often appear together, especially in baked goods. "Muffins are bready and brown and often have raisins in them, so they look very healthy, but they can contain as much fat as you'd want in an entire meal," says Susan Kayman, Dr.P.H., R.D., a nutrition consultant with the Kaiser Permanente Medical Group in Oakland, California. When in doubt about whether you're eating

• •

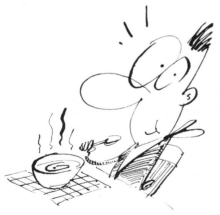

Soup Tames
the Appetite

You're so famished that you skip the menu and head straight for the all-you-can-eat buffet. Trouble is, usually when you are *that* hungry, you eat too fast and too much, which leaves you feeling as sluggish as a walrus. To avoid gorging yourself, start your meal with a bowl of soup. In a study at Johns Hopkins University, a tomato soup appetizer reduced calorie consumption over the course of an entire meal by 25 percent, compared with a cheese-and-crackers appetizer. That may be because soup takes up more space in the stomach, making you feel full.

mainly fat or carbohydrates, the litmus test is to put the food on a paper napkin, she says. "Anything that leaves a grease stain is fatty."

High-fat foods that can masquerade as low-fat ones include:

■ Crackers. They look wholesome, but some are as fatty as potato chips. Slathering on cheese spread makes them even worse. Lower-fat alternatives include Ry-Krisp or melba toast.

■ Croissants. Don't let a filling of, say, broccoli fool you. Croissants were invented by the French, after all, and every one of those thin layers of pastry is made with a fresh coating of butter.

■ Baked potatoes. On their own, potatoes are excellent sources of carbohydrates, but heaps of butter or sour cream tell another story. Choose instead toppings such as yogurt, salsa or low-fat cottage cheese.

■ Microwave popcorn (or any kind of popcorn you don't air-pop yourself). Most use a heavy dose of oil as part of their preparation.

2. You need to cut calories drastically to lose weight. Not really. When you cut back too hard on your calories, the body goes into a conservation mode in which your metabolism—the rate at which the body's calorie-burning machinery turns over—switches to a slower idle. That actually decreases your ability to lose weight.

To keep your body revving, the experts advise that you drop your total calorie intake only a little while adjusting the fuel mix. "Cut back just on fat, and you can practically eat the same number of calories and still lose weight," says Kim Galeaz Gioe, R.D., spokesperson for the American Dietetic Association. In a study at Cornell University, people who got 25 percent of their calories from fat (as opposed to the 38 percent typical for most men) but ate as much as they wanted of other types of food lost an average of a half-pound per week.

3. Only drastic diets work. We'll grant that if you eat nothing but grapefruit morning, noon and night, you will lose weight. But if you're considering a diet like this, we suggest you look in the mirror and say these words out loud: "I will never in my life eat anything but grapefruit again."

Right. The problem with extreme diets is that they ignore reality—a certain undeniable craving for roast beef that is bound to set in midway through a grapefruit diet. And once you go back to your old eating ways, you'll quickly gain the pounds back.

To take weight off and keep it off, experts instead advise making small, gradual changes you can live with. We're talking changes so innocuous that it won't seem like you've started a diet at all.

When ordering fast food, for example, get the same burger but tell them to leave off the cheese. You'll save 100 calories per meal, more than half of them from fat. Get your breakfast sandwich on a bagel instead of a fattier croissant and save 200 calories. Use low-fat mayonnaise and "lite" margarines in a tub; most taste as good but have half the fat of regular products. (Despite recent reports on the health hazards of margarine, "lite" tub margarines are still a much better option than butter.) Avoid fatty salad toppings such as eggs, olives and regular dressing. Drink 1 percent milk instead of 2 percent or whole milk. "Don't think you're limited to skim," says Gioe. "One percent is perfectly consistent with USDA (U.S. Department of Agriculture) guidelines for a low-fat diet."

In one study at Indiana University, people who bought low-fat dairy and meat products, put fewer fatty extras on their foods and ate fewer fried foods easily dropped the percentage of fat in their diets from 39 to 27 percent.

4. You have to give up favorite foods. You don't. In fact, you can eat anything you want. "The minute you say 'I can't' or 'I shouldn't,' you're setting yourself up for disaster," Gioe says. "Instead, you need to turn it around and ask 'How can I squeeze in my favorite high-fat foods and still lose weight?' "

Depriving yourself of pleasure from food isn't fun, and it doesn't work. "There's something called the abstinence violation effect, which says that if you insist on completely avoiding something, human nature makes it likely that you'll break your resolution," Dr. Kayman says. "Then you tell yourself you've blown it and simply give up. It's much better to allow yourself enjoyable choices now and then, which makes the real issue how much you have and how often."

Take, for example, ice cream, rated in a survey as the favorite dessert among men. You could have it three times a week as part of a low-fat diet, as long as you follow one of two guidelines: either have small, half-cup portions of the real thing or have larger, one-cup helpings of low-fat varieties or frozen yogurt.

Red meat is another food that can readily be part of a healthy diet if you eat small portions once or twice a week. Choosing a lean cut allows you to eat bigger portions. Here's a simple rule: Anything with the words "round" or "loin" is low-fat. Sirloin, tenderloin and eye of round, for example, all

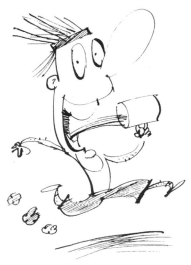

Take a Performance Break

Drinking strong coffee before a race may help you shave those last few stubborn minutes off your personal best for a marathon, suggest Canadian studies. In one experiment, distance runners took caffeine tablets (roughly equal to three mugs of strong coffee) one hour before running or cycling until exhaustion. Running endurance increased from an average 49 minutes to 71 minutes, and cycling endurance increased from 39 minutes to 59 minutes. The latest word is that the equivalent of one or two mugs of strong coffee may work just as well, says Terry Graham, Ph.D., who coauthored the studies with Lawrence Spriet, Ph.D. Dr. Graham and Dr. Spriet are associate professors of physiology at the University of Guelph in Guelph, Ontario. "Caffeine causes the body to burn more fat for energy, sparing the carbohydrates stored in the muscles for a longer time," Dr. Graham says. "But you'd be crazy to try this during a race if you haven't tried it in practice. Some athletes performed worse after taking caffeine."

come from muscular, lean parts of a cow. Rib eye and prime rib, by contrast, come from softer, fattier parts, and you should eat less of them.

5. You shouldn't snack. The right kinds of snacks can actually help you lose weight.

The important thing is to take control of your snack supply to make sure that it's low in fat. You can't rely on standard fare from office vending machines or company caterers, which provide ample selections of just the things you want to avoid: high-fat candy bars, snack chips and rich doughnuts and pastries. Instead, Dr. Kayman suggests you bring a bag filled with a variety of foods you can nosh on throughout the day. Fruits such as apples and bananas are good choices, as are bagels with jam or jelly and small cans of vegetable juice. Snacking on low-fat, energy-rich foods like these will keep you from becoming too hungry and overeating at mealtimes.

In addition, the wide variety of low-fat foods being packaged these days has suddenly made sweets acceptable as snacks. "I used to eat a brownie only as a special treat, not more than once a month," Gioe says. "Now I can have a huge one almost every day, thanks to low-fat mixes."

6. When you overeat, it's because you're hungry. Hunger has nothing to do with it. We overeat for emotional reasons, according to Maria Simonson, Ph.D., Sc.D., director of the health, weight and stress clinic at Johns Hopkins Medical Institutions in Baltimore. If you know your emotional triggers, you'll also eat better.

"One of the major reasons is stress," she says. "Stress makes you eat more quickly than anything else." And the foods you want to eat under stress are more likely to be fatty, pleasurable things that are soft or creamy.

These cravings aren't commands from the body, however. Nor will they continue to torment you until you give in. In fact, they can change as quickly as the emotions that drive them. Cravings follow a predictable curve, researchers found: They build, peak, then subside. The best way to foil a craving is to take your mind off it, preferably by doing something incompatible with eating, such as going for a walk.

7. Burning fat demands intense exercise. Not true. Most any exercise burns fat. According to Janet Walberg-

Rankin, Ph.D., associate professor of exercise physiology at Virginia Polytechnic Institute and State University, you can lose a pound a week just by ratcheting your activity level up a notch or two. By this she means things such as walking, chopping wood, mowing the lawn, cleaning the basement or climbing stairs.

It used to be thought that you needed standard three-times-a-week regimens of intense workouts to pare away pounds. Such workouts are important for improving cardiovascular fitness, but fat burning takes place at lower intensity levels, says Bryant Stamford, Ph.D., professor of allied health at the University of Louisville. "The exercise doesn't have to be a killer for weight loss," he says.

Intensity is a trade-off, Dr. Stamford says. The harder you work, the more you'll burn, but if you find hard exercise unpleasant, you won't stick with it. Lighter exercise, he finds, pays higher dividends in the long run because it's more easily sustained.

8. Aerobic exercise is better than lifting weights. You'll burn more fat *during* an aerobic workout than you will doing a set of weights, but the benefits from aerobics end shortly after exercising. Strength training, on the other hand, keeps the flab-torching flame alive long after the workout is over. "Weight training is like a salary," Dr. Stamford says. "Aerobics is like a bonus."

It all has to do with how efficiently your metabolism burns fat. Weight lifting builds muscle fast, and muscle is the most metabolically supercharged tissue in the body. "If you raise your metabolic rate even a fraction, it's multiplied by 60 minutes, 24 hours a day," Dr. Stamford says. "You lose weight just from being alive."

He recommends a weight workout that hits all the major muscle groups. Whether you use machines or free weights makes no difference. Aim for two sets of 12 repetitions per exercise. If you can do 12 reps without too much strain, add enough weight to make the last few lifts difficult.

The best part of all this is that with experts now advocating occasional splurges, you'll never have to make another resolution about what you eat. In a word, enjoy.

—Richard Laliberte

Part 3

MEN AT EASE

Unwind at Last!

Since you're already so good at working hard,
here are 21 workaholic-proof ways to relax.

• • • • • • • • • • • • • • • • • •

MOST MEN DON'T PUT a high value on relaxation. We
score ourselves on measurable things such as achievement
and pay, not emotional tranquility. "Men tend to look at
relaxing as a waste of time," says Paul J. Rosch, M.D., president of the American Institute of Stress in Yonkers, New
York. "We feel guilty if we aren't productive."

"We've been taught to always do and perform, to act like
Superman," adds Keith Sedlacek, M.D., medical director of

the Stress Regulation Institute in New York City. "Of course, we all know what happened to Superman. . . ."

Okay, we know what you're thinking: "Yeah, I have a little trouble unwinding, but it isn't going to kill me." Well, indirectly, it could. Considered by experts to be the major health problem facing men today, stress has been linked to heart disease, high blood pressure, stroke, cancer and other illnesses—even impotence. Up to 90 percent of all visits to doctors are for stress-related disorders, according to the American Institute of Stress.

Stress often surfaces as a health problem in men because men wait too long to do something about it. Only 20 percent of the people enrolled in a typical stress management program are males, says Joan Borysenko, Ph.D., president of Mind-Body Health Sciences in Boulder, Colorado. "Men take longer than women to realize that they are in trouble," she says. Learning to unwind is not easy, particularly if you're the hard-driving, achievement-oriented type. "It takes effort— that's the paradox," says Allen Elkin, Ph.D., director of the Stress Management and Counseling Center in New York City. "You have to find what'll do the job for you."

There are a number of basic rules for keeping from getting wound too tight. The first is to add balance to your life. Make a special attempt to seek out leisure activities that are different from your work. "Our bodies require variety and change," says Dr. Sedlacek. "We have to shift gears, readjust our speed, or our nervous systems will keep racing right into the next day." An accountant or lawyer who spends his week in analytic, left-brain pursuits might find relaxation in chopping wood, gardening, building a deck or tinkering with a car engine. In fact, almost any white-collar type would benefit from manual labor of some kind.

The second rule is to work up a sweat once in a while. Research by Robert Thayer, Ph.D., a professor of psychology at California State University, shows that 30 minutes of intense aerobic exercise immediately reduces body tension— and does it more effectively than moderate exercise such as walking. New research at Hofstra University has also found that weight lifting counters anxiety and depression and boosts self-esteem as well as or better than aerobic exercise.

The third rule is that whatever you choose as a relaxation break, it has to be relaxing *to you*. "If someone tells you to tie trout flies and you find it boring as hell, you'll actually add to your stress," warns Dr. Rosch.

Finally, you've got to carve little breaks into your schedule. "You need to put together a relaxation package, a set of techniques that'll calm you down," says Dr. Elkin.

Here are some ideas to try.

Pad your schedule. "Realize that nearly everything will take longer than you anticipate," says Richard Swenson, M.D., author of *Margin: How to Create the Emotional, Physical, Financial and Time Reserves You Need.* By allotting yourself enough time to accomplish a task, you cut back on anxiety. In general, if meeting deadlines is a problem, always give yourself 20 percent more time than you think you need to do the task.

Carry a canteen. Keep a plastic bottle of water at your

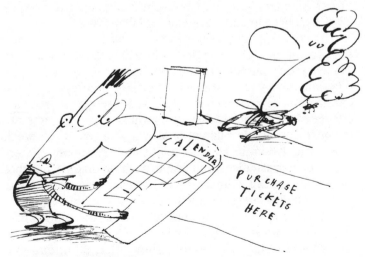

Bargain Travel Days

A travel tip: More discount fares are available for flights on Tuesday and Wednesday, at midday or late evening. The most expensive flights are usually Mondays and Fridays—particularly during the morning and evening rush hours.

desk and drink often. When you are under stress, you sweat more; and then, of course, there's your dry mouth. You'll feel better if you hydrate your high anxiety.

Kill the ump. You can blow off your emotions at a ball game and get some of the tension out of your system, says Roger Thies, Ph.D., associate professor of physiology at the University of Oklahoma Health Sciences Center. "By yelling something really nasty, you almost make a joke of it, and you may head off that adrenaline squirt on your heart." (Just make sure the drunken guy in front of you isn't rooting for the other team.) Other places to let off steam: sports bars, pep rallies, political conventions. Places not to let off steam: church services, snow-covered cliffs, your father-in-law's house.

Practice your snorkeling. Want to really relax your muscles? Soak in a hot tub. To get the most relaxation from a hot bath, soak for 15 minutes in water that's just a few degrees warmer than your body temperature, about 100° to 101°F. But be careful: Longer soaks in warmer water can actually lower your blood pressure too much.

Get a grip. Keep a hand exerciser or a tennis ball in your desk and give it a few squeezes during tense times. "When stress shoots adrenaline into the bloodstream, that calls for muscle action," says Roger Cady, M.D., medical director of the Shealy Institute for Comprehensive Health Care in Springfield, Missouri. "Squeezing something provides a release that satisfies our bodies' fight-or-flee response."

Serve soup, live longer. Be a volunteer. Isolation only magnifies your worries. Helping others will give you a sense of accomplishment and self-respect—and remind you that relatively speaking, your own troubles don't amount to a hill of beans in this world. Here's an added benefit: Self-sacrifice may help you live longer. A ten-year University of Michigan study found that the death rate was twice as high in men who did no volunteer work as in men who volunteered their time at least once a week.

Sit up straight. A good upright posture improves breathing and increases blood flow to the brain. We often slouch when stressed, which restricts breathing and blood flow and can magnify feelings of helplessness.

Pop a bubble. A recent study found that students were able to reduce their feelings of tension by popping two sheets of those plastic air capsules used in packaging. "Now we know why people hoard those things," says Kathy M. Dillon, Ph.D., a professor of psychology at Western New England College and the author of the study.

Trade in the Jag for a Hyundai. Living beyond your means can actually make you sick. A researcher at the University of Alabama studied British census data of 8,000 households and found that families that tried to maintain a lifestyle they couldn't afford were likely to have health problems.

Carry a humor first-aid kit. We could cite you chapter and verse on the value of humor in the workplace. Past studies have shown that stress-fighting brain chemicals are released when you laugh. Some experts believe all it takes is a smile to ignite a positive mood. Unfortunately, repeating Jay Leno's monologue at the watercooler every morning gets tired pretty fast, especially if you have a boss who's prone to say things like "Time is money." For some fresh ideas that won't stunt your career growth, send a self-addressed envelope with 75 cents postage to: The Humor Project, 110 Spring Street, Saratoga Springs, NY 12866.

Hold your breath. This technique should help you to relax in 30 seconds. Take a deep breath and keep it in. Holding palm to palm, press your fingers together. Wait 5 seconds, then slowly exhale through your lips while letting your hands relax. Do this five or six times until you unwind.

Smell the apples. Keeping a green apple on your desk may calm your nerves. A recent study found that men doing math problems under time pressure were less stressed if they were exposed to the scent of green apples. There's evidence that the scent of vanilla may also induce relaxation in men, says Alan R. Hirsch, M.D., neurologic director of the Smell and Taste Treatment and Research Foundation in Chicago.

Dare to be dull. Join the International Dull Men's Club. "We are regular guys who aren't hyper, self-absorbed or pushy," says president Joe Troise. "When you can say 'It's okay to be dull,' it takes a lot of life's pressures off." For a $5 membership fee, you get a license that certifies you as a dull person, plus some infrequent newsletters. The address: 300 Napa Street, #10, Sausalito, CA 94965.

Jog your brain. In one study, students who ran twice a week for 20 minutes scored higher on creativity tests than did students who were required to sit through lectures. Researchers say running induces a relaxed-brain state, where thoughts are thrown together randomly and new ideas often emerge. We say, get the entire cast of "Saturday Night Live" some new Nikes.

Rubberneck. When you get wound too tight, often the first place you feel it is your neck. Try this four-way neck release recommended by former world-class track and field athlete Greg Herzog in his book *The 15-Minute Executive Stress-Relief Program.* (Repeat each exercise three times.)

1. Reach with your right hand over your head and behind your left ear, grasping your neck with your fingers. Pull your head gently toward your right shoulder.

2. Do the same exercise, but this time use your left hand to pull your head toward your left shoulder.

3. Clasp your hands behind your head with your elbows flared and your head bowed toward your chest. Relax in this

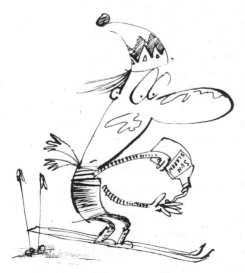

Cover Your Nose

Skiers who take medication may need to cover their noses, cheeks and ears with a strong sunscreen before hitting the slopes. According to the Food and Drug Administration, certain common medications may increase skin sensitivity to ultraviolet rays. The drugs include antihistamines, ibuprofen and tetracyclines as well as certain tranquilizers such as Trilafon and Stelazine.

position for 30 seconds. Then while pulling down with your hands, slowly push your head back until you are looking at the ceiling.

4. Place the palm of your left hand on your forehead with the bottom of your palm at the bridge of your nose. Hold your right arm across your body so that you can rest your left elbow on your right wrist. Now push against your left palm with your forehead while keeping your right arm locked. Switch hands and repeat.

Find your mantra. If your idea of meditation is that blank feeling you get paying bills every month, consider that guys who tune out the world for 20 minutes twice a day may live longer. In a study, meditators had levels of a good-for-you type of hormone that were comparable to those of nonmeditators five to ten years younger, says Jay Glaser, M.D., medical director of Maharishi Ayur-Veda Health Center in Lancaster, Massachusetts. To find a teacher in your area, call (800) 843-8332.

Tune out—have a potato. If you want to unwind at the end of the day, eat a meal high in carbohydrates, says Judith Wurtman, Ph.D., a researcher at the Massachusetts Institute of Technology and author of *Managing Your Mind and Mood through Food.* Carbohydrates trigger the brain chemical serotonin, which soothes you. Good carbohydrate foods include rice, pasta, potatoes, breads, air-popped popcorn and low-calorie cookies. Dr. Wurtman says just 1½ ounces of carbohydrates is enough to relieve the anxiety of a stressful day.

Tune in—have a steak. It's no help unwinding if you're feeling sluggish and unalert. Dr. Wurtman suggests a high-protein lunch of lean meat, fish or poultry to prevent the afternoon blahs. Protein is loaded with tyrosine, an amino acid that has been shown to boost mental performance in the face of stress.

Make your kids sign out. It's impossible to unwind if you are spending two hours worrying about kids who took off before you got home and didn't leave a forwarding address. Stick a message board and an erasable marker on the refrigerator and tell your kids to note where they went and a phone number where they can be reached. Just pray it never reads "Went to visit the Buttafuocos."

Don't track dirt in. When you get home from work, avoid the temptation to bitch about your workday. Home should be a sanctuary. "Men tend to recount the stresses of the day, and all that does is contaminate their homes," says Neil Fiore, Ph.D., a Berkeley, California, psychologist and author of *The Road Back to Health*. Instead, set aside ten minutes or so of quiet time to put the workday behind you before you try to leap into your loving-father-and-husband routine.

Quit the bowling league. Look at your life. Are you doing too much? If you're on the company softball team, coaching Little League, volunteering on a church committee, chauffeuring kids to piano lessons and Girl Scout outings and you don't have a weeknight free, you're choking on more than you can chew. "Prune your activity branches," suggests Dr. Swenson. Decide what gives you the most pleasure and do only those things.

—Jeffrey Csatari

A Beginner's Guide to Scuba Diving

Diving is as close as you can get to unaided flight— and it's safer than baseball!

● ● ● ● ● ● ● ● ● ● ● ● ● ● ● ● ● ●

IT ISN'T OFTEN YOU WAKE UP on the bottom of the ocean. But there I was. Somewhere above on the busy island of St. Croix, people were making coffee and getting into the daily grind. A quarter-mile offshore and 60 feet below the surface, I might as well have been on the dark side of the moon. No television, no radio, no newspaper intruded on my newfound and wholly aquatic reality. A mutton snapper hovered just outside my window, pondering me as I pondered my sit-

● ●

GETTING STARTED

For information on diving retailers, check your Yellow Pages under "Diving." To get information on diving instruction in your area or abroad, check with:

■ National Association of Scuba Diving Schools, 8099 Indiana Avenue, Riverside, CA 92504; (800) 735-3483.

■ National Association of Underwater Instructors, 4650 Arrow Highway, Suite F-1, Montclair, CA 91763; (800) 553-6284, ext. 209.

■ Professional Association of Diving Instructors, 1251 East Dyer Road, #100, Santa Ana, CA 92705.

■ Professional Diving Instructors Corporation International, 1554 Gardner Avenue, Scranton, PA 18505.

■ Scuba Schools International, 2619 Canton Court, Fort Collins, CO 80525; (800) 892-2702.

WHAT IT COSTS

You can sign up for a full certification course at your local dive retail store for $100 to $150. Included in the cost is use of a

● ●

uation. The day before, I had been principally a land animal, bound by evolutionary necessity to the world of light and air. This day, in a laboratory on the bottom of Salt River Canyon in the Caribbean, I felt closer kinship to the marine world. My front door was a round hatch connecting the lab's dry living quarters with the open ocean. Going for a stroll meant slipping into a scuba tank and stroking along the wall of the canyon to the sheer coral cliff a few hundred yards seaward.

I strolled.

As I approached the edge, the solid ground began to give way. But the water held me up, and I was in no danger of falling. Pushing myself gently beyond the lip, I soared out over the cliff. At this spot, the sea floor plunges in one shot from 100 feet to a depth of almost two miles, twice as deep as the Grand Canyon.

regulator, a weight belt (to keep you from floating to the surface), a buoyancy compensator (to keep the weighted you from sinking to the bottom) and tanks. Most courses will require you to buy a mask ($40 to $80), fins ($40 to $100) and snorkel ($10 to $20), plus a textbook and a set of dive tables ($25 to $40) that show how long you can safely stay at a specific depth. All told, you can figure a total of about $300 to become amphibious.

Once you're certified, you don't need to buy any more equipment than the mask, fins and snorkel. You can rent the regulator, weight belt, buoyancy compensator and tanks at just about any dive site in the world. Many beginners do, however, invest in a regulator ($200 to $500) and a buoyancy compensator ($200 to $400).

Other good investments for those who are beginning to get serious about diving include a dive computer ($350 to $750), which keeps track of your tank pressure, depth, time in the water and time remaining before surfacing; gloves ($30 to $50); wet suit ($150 to $500); dive light ($30 to $100); and booties ($25 to $50).

Facing toward the wall, I watched psychedelic-colored parrot fish hunt for breakfast among clumps of coral festooned with human-size sponges glowing purple in the filtered morning light. Somewhere deep in my subconscious, it all connected. Maybe with another age. Maybe with an age to come.

"This," I thought, "is living."

TAKE OFF UNDERWATER

Of course, I eventually had to leave the lab and come ashore. (Eventually, the lab did, too—it's now gathering dust on the floor of the Smithsonian.) But I still revisit the submarine world whenever I can. Diving is as close as you can get to unaided flight. It is rappelling without ropes; flying without wings. And while most land animals have learned to fear humans, most aquatic ones don't, allowing the most amazing up-close-and-personal interaction with wildlife. Swimming with a Yugo-size sea turtle or being buzzed by a pod of dol-phins—sleek gray torpedoes flashing by as if to mock the clumsy, lumbering fools from above—is an experience you can't easily forget.

It's also an experience you can't have unless you learn to dive. That means getting certified, known in the biz as "getting your C-card." The card proves to dive boat operators you've completed an approved educational course. You can't make a dive from a boat, or even get scuba tanks filled with air, without flashing the card.

Remember the 1960s TV series "Sea Hunt"? Lloyd Bridges played underwater detective Mike Nelson, who could barely manage to take a bath without getting involved in some sort of life-threatening scrape. A steady diet of that during your impressionable years may have left you with the idea that diving is riskier than it is.

Don't get me wrong: There's plenty of challenge left. But diving is not just for daredevils anymore. In fact, recre-ational scuba diving has a lower incidence of injury than American football, baseball, waterskiing, soccer, volleyball, racquetball, tennis and swimming, according to Drew Richardson, director of training for the Professional Association of Diving Instructors.

An estimated four million Americans have C-cards, with 300,000 joining them each year. Three-quarters are men, although diving couples are increasingly common. And with demographics hovering in the same stratospheric neighbor-hood as golf and sailing, the sport has grown unquestion-ably chic.

IT'S EASIER THAN YOU THINK

Another misconception about scuba: People often mis-takenly assume that the certification program is a test of Herculean proportions. Here's a quick qualification drill: Fill a bathtub with water. Get in. Hold your nose. Duck your head under. No panic? Fine, you'll do.

Diving isn't the most physically demanding activity. All it requires is good general health and some stamina. Before you begin a certification course, you'll have to get a doctor's okay that you're fit. Chronic asthma, emphysema, diabetes requiring drugs or insulin and a history of seizures are definite disqualifiers. Less common conditions, such as severe or chronic ear, sinus or heart problems, may or may not keep you from diving. A doctor familiar with diving medicine is your best bet for a precourse checkup. If you can't find one in your area, you can request information on physicians who are trained or knowledgeable in diving medicine from the Undersea and Hyperbaric Medical Society, 9650 Rockville Pike, Bethesda, MD 20814, or the Divers Alert Network at Duke University, 3100 Tower Boulevard, Suite 1300, Durham, NC 27707.

Your scuba classes will progress in two phases—classroom instruction and pool work—for a total of 16 to 20 hours. Commonly, classes are offered two nights a week, 2 hours per class, with the pool and classroom sessions extending over four or five weeks. Some instructors also

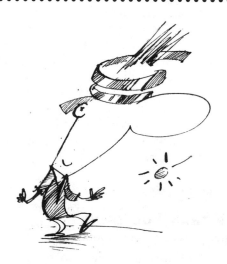

Wraparound Sun Protection

Just wearing a good pair of regular sunglasses isn't always enough to protect your eyes from the harmful effects of the sun. Australian researchers say you're better off wearing wraparound shades to keep the sun's rays out. Exposure to sunlight has been implicated in a number of eye disorders, including cataracts.

offer intensive weekend courses, with classes meeting 8 hours per day but finishing up in two weekends.

However it's structured, at the end of the term you'll be given a simple written test to confirm for the instructor that you weren't dozing off during the most important stuff. Which is entirely possible, since most of the classroom part has to do with atmospheric pressure. You need to know about this because as you go deeper in the water, the pressure on your body increases. This affects the pressure of the air your regulator delivers to your mouthpiece, and for deep dives, it also affects the amounts of nitrogen and oxygen that are pressed into your blood. Going too deep for too long, and returning to the surface suddenly, can make the nitrogen in your blood fizz right out, just like taking the cap off a bottle of cola after you shake it. This is called decompression sickness, or the bends, and it's not good for you, to put it mildly.

Despite the fact that the risk of getting the bends provides the dramatic high point for practically every Jacques Cousteau special, the actual incidence is low. According to Karen Corson, a diving epidemiologist with Divers Alert Network, only about 4 divers in 10,000 will experience decompression sickness. Still, you've got to learn about it, so you don't make a stupid mistake. You'll also learn how to travel under the ocean without harming the environment, how to interact—or how to avoid interacting—with the animals and other useful skills.

NOW THE FUN STARTS

Most divers find the pool instruction much more fun. Here's where you get to strap on a tank, get down and actually breathe underwater. You'll learn how to assemble your gear and use the various pieces, how to swim efficiently underwater with fins, how to flush water out of your mask should it leak (not nearly as difficult as it sounds) and a variety of safety procedures.

After your pool and classroom sessions are finished, you'll make about four open-water dives with your instructor. These are for you to practice the skills you learned in class. You'll have an instructor present to help you with anything you haven't quite mastered. On the first open-water dive, you'll be called on to demonstrate some of the skills, such as flooding your mask and then clearing it of water. In land-locked areas, these dives are often held in lakes, quarries or springs. In coastal areas, they're done in the ocean.

As with the written test, the purpose of the checkout dives isn't to wash you out or disqualify you but to help the instructor judge whether you're ready to dive without super-

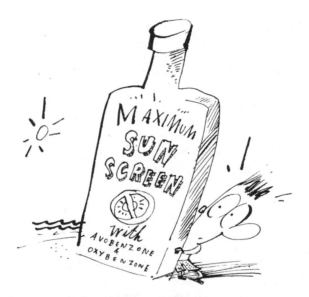

Beaches and Cream

Slathering on an SPF (sun protection factor) 15 sunscreen won't keep all the sun's ultraviolet rays away from your sensitive flesh. While most sunscreens do a great job of blocking out the ultraviolet B (UVB) rays, they still allow some of the ultraviolet A (UVA) variety to sneak through. But the Food and Drug Administration recently approved a new combination of sunscreen ingredients, avobenzone and oxybenzone, that absorbs the most UVA radiation yet. The two are found in Shade UVAGuard, a PABA-free sunscreen made by Schering-Plough. A four-ounce bottle of the lotion, which also screens out UVB rays, costs about $10.

vision and to help you feel safe and comfortable in the water.

In some cases, students complete their classroom work at home, then book a trip to an area with clear, warm water, such as the Caribbean, to do their open-water dives. In this case, your instructor will write a letter confirming that you've completed your classroom instruction. Most dive resorts have instructors on staff who will gladly do the checkout dives with you for a small fee.

If you want to, you can book a trip to a resort and get certified there. Costs vary widely, but $250 is a common figure, and that usually includes the rental of all gear (including mask, fins and snorkel) and the cost of the checkout dives. Add airfare and accommodations, and it can be a pricey option. It may be a good one, however. The advantage is that you learn how to dive in a place with warm, clear water and colorful coral reefs. The disadvantage, of course, is that you end up spending a lot of time—16 hours or more—indoors during your vacation.

Still another option is taking a noncertification resort course. Most dive resorts offer these. You spend about four hours preparing in the classroom, then go on a real dive that same day under the supervision of an instructor. It's the quickest way to get in the water and see whether you like it. Again, prices vary, but the cost should be in the range of $125. The disadvantage here is that after you spend the money and the time, you don't have a C-card to show for it. If you find you want to pursue diving, you'll still need to take a full course to get certified.

Okay, let's say you've gotten this far and you're still asking "Why? What's the big deal about diving?" For a lot of us, the answer is "Because it's there." You can't know the ocean by sailing on top of it. That's like exploring a forest from an airliner. You have to get down amongst the coral. You have to be close enough to see the rainbow in a catfish whisker, to feel the silky underbelly of a stingray.

IT'S IN OUR GENES

Diving is the only sport to which we have a genetically programmed predisposition, by the way, a relic of our evolution from sea creatures. The mammalian diving reflex kicks in as water pressure on the body increases and water temperature drops. To conserve oxygen, the heart rate slows, and blood is rerouted from the extremities to the brain. While your first dive will doubtless make your heart race and your senses reel, with time diving becomes a trancelike, almost transcendental experience. Remote as we are from our aquatic ancestors, the mark of the sea is still upon us.

—*Steve Blount*

Next Stop: France!
*Who needs tile and chlorine when there
are big, bad oceans to swim?*

• • • • • • • • • • • • • • • • •

MY FATHER COULDN'T DO a flip turn, and neither can I. He was never on a swim team, and he didn't even have a real kick. My father was an ocean swimmer, and I, like him, love the open water. He was raised in Atlantic City and loves to tell stories about midnight swims through inky waves around the glittering Steel Pier. One night he swam a half-mile out to the end of the famous pier, made his way up a ladder, sprinted across the glowing dance floor there and dived into the heaving swells on the other side. He was no pool swimmer; he was a water man. All winter I pine for the ocean, where a swim isn't just a workout, it's an adventure. Who wants to slog back and forth the length of a pool like a goldfish in a bowl when you could actually go somewhere with your stroke? Who wants to look at the tile on the bottom of a swimming pool when with each breath, with each twist of your head, you could witness the scrolling spectacle of lofty sky, distant beach, frothy surface and briny depths?

Near Montauk Point, on the eastern tip of Long Island, there's a mile-wide arc of beach popular with surfers. Visiting for the day last September, I decided to take a swim alone. There had been a hurricane the week before, but now

● ●

THE ART OF
OCEAN SWIMMING

Ocean swimming requires minimal equipment: Any racing-style suit and a pair of goggles will do. Spend a little extra money for the tinted, UV-protective kind, because these will cut glare as well as keep water out of your eyes.

A lot of ocean swimmers swear by flippers. These certainly get you around faster, and the word is they give your legs a better workout.

At an unfamiliar beach, you should watch the water carefully, gauge the sweep from left to right, find out about the tides and the bottom. You should know if there are sandbars or reefs beyond the shore break. It's always a good idea to query a local about conditions—a lifeguard, a surfer, even a fisherman.

There are spots in the ocean where the undertow is stronger, where underwater cuts in the sandbars cause the water to run out. Lifeguards call them rip currents. From the land you can see that the water in a rip is lighter and more bubbly than the water on both sides. The rip generally sucks out to sea for a few hundred yards and then stops pulling. If you find yourself in a rip, swim parallel with the beach until you are out of its grasp, then head in.

Entrance is important. A shore break can slap you upside your head, take you over the falls and break your bones. Watch the wave patterns. Stand on the beach for 20 minutes if you have to. Be prepared to spend the whole day on the beach if things don't look right. When you enter, keep your body sideways, so the break can't get a full hit on you. If the ocean is really pumping, as you dive under the waves dig your fingers in the sand to avoid being pulled back. Exiting the water in a spot where there is a rowdy shore break can be dangerous. Just because you're ready to come ashore, don't assume the ocean is ready to let you leave. Tread water beyond the breaker line with the same patience you employed on the beach. And as you come ashore, never turn your back on the break. Keep looking over your shoulder; you never know when some monster wave might be gaining on you.

● ●

the sparkling green ocean lifted and reared gently in the morning sun. Four-foot waves wrapped around the point beyond a small jetty. I left my clothes on the beach close to the rocks and jogged about a mile down the beach to a spot where three long poles protruded from the wind-flattened gray sand.

The run warmed me up, and I knew the cool September seawater would be delicious on my skin. I ducked under the shore break, porpoised three times and stroked out into the water. I chose my angle across the cove and started to reach and pull. With each breath, as my eyes broke the surface, I saw the sun-dappled ocean slipping by, framed by the sand and looming cliffs. I alternated my breaths from left to right. On one side, I saw the cliffs; on the other, the endless, open sea. I felt the chill blast of an icy current from below and then the warm touch of a sheath of sun-warmed surface water. The sensation of running through a forest is fine, but swimming alone across a painted ocean is exquisite.

KNOW WHAT YOU'RE DOING

Of course, you have to know what you're doing. When I was a teenager frolicking in storm surf with my knockabout buddies, we used to remind ourselves to respect the Big O. But "respect" is much too puny a word to use for the level of attention that must be paid the ocean. Besides healthy fear, ocean swimming demands its own technique.

Bob Kolonkowski, professional lifeguard and president of the Jones Beach chapter of the United States Lifesaving Association, describes the ocean stroke: "Both the kick and the arm motion can be different in the ocean. Because salt water is more buoyant, you float higher. For that reason, the kick is less propulsive than in fresh water. Also, your arm recovery must be higher, so you'll clear the irregular surface. You want to be able to break the surface and look straight ahead every several strokes to correct your direction and keep on course."

According to Kolonkowski, there should be a much greater emphasis on the arm stroke in the ocean. "You have to be able to vary your stroke," he says. "You rely on a shorter stroke to lift yourself out of choppy water, and you use that same short pull to punch through waves when you're heading out."

Direction's important, too. A lot of times you swim out and around something (a buoy, for instance), and you can get thrown off course and end up way down the beach. "When you are swimming in the ocean," Kolonkowski advises, "you should pick out a building or a natural landmark and use it as a guide."

A good ocean swimmer must also develop the technique of breathing on both the left and right sides. You want to be able to sight your marker on one side and still watch the incoming waves on the other. Another trick is to take your breaths on the sunny side. This can sometimes warm your body and your spirits on those cold-water swims.

NEVER SWIM BLIND—OR ALONE

An experienced water man knows never to plunge into unfamiliar water. And he keeps in mind a rule so old it sounds like an empty threat: Don't swim alone.

For example: that Montauk swim I was telling you about? I swam my heart out. After a half-hour, I raised my head to check the location of the jetty. I was a little farther out than I had intended, but I was almost parallel with the gray-green stone jetty. I was pleasantly tired. Satisfied.

I dug my left arm into the water and wheeled toward the shore. I felt the surge and draw of the swells now. As I pulled and breathed, I had to be more careful of the water level—a couple of times I swallowed brine. I almost laughed

• •

Treat Your Stomach Gingerly

Every time you go deep-sea fishing with your buddies, you end up chumming the tarpon with your breakfast. Seasickness pills make you drowsy, but there may be a better way. Next time you step on a boat, try sucking on some ginger. Studies have demonstrated that ginger can help combat nausea, says Varro E. Tyler, Ph.D., professor of pharmacognosy at Purdue University. Whole gingerroot is most effective, but a tastier alternative, crystallized ginger candy, should work as well. You can buy it at Asian grocery stores.

to myself. The water was clean and salty. To put the cap on my workout, I sped up my stroke and started to breathe every other stroke. I labored mightily, sucked in air and blew it back in the frothy sea. Almost spent, I raised my head up, ready to walk ashore.

I was stunned. I was still a hundred yards out. In three minutes of hard swimming, I hadn't moved ten feet.

I stripped my goggles from my face and looked at the shore again. My pile of clothes was a tiny speck on the distant sand. As the ocean rose and fell around me, I began to lose sight of the beach altogether.

I planed myself in the water and began to pull and kick. After a minute, I looked up again. The shore was still a hundred yards away, and the panic was born. My first impulse was to throw off my new goggles as if they were casting a spell, giving me incorrect bearings. But it wasn't my eyes that were troubling me. It was my judgment.

I SHOULD HAVE KNOWN BETTER

I should have known better, much better. I should have known that the jetty might create a suck. And I should have known not to be in the water by myself.

I think my dreamy state of mind brought on by the solitude and the caress of the water had something to do with my rapid descent into panic. If I had been thinking, I would have drifted 30 or 40 yards to the right or left, rested for a minute and cruised into shore out of the grip of the undertow.

Instead, I fought the ocean.

This time I had no illusions about my progress. I knew I would have to power like a madman for two or three minutes. At last, my left hand scraped the blessed bottom. I crawled up on the shore and sprawled on the beach, my limbs pumped with air, like balloons. The gulls floating above were the only witnesses to my folly. I had always believed myself to be drown-proof. Not anymore.

Ocean swimming is a glorious sport, an unparalleled method of staying in shape, but you can't just dive in and start stroking. You can't be just a swimmer. You have to be a water man.

—Greg Donaldson

A Sportsman's Guide to Winning at Everything

Think winning isn't everything? Well, this chapter is for men who aren't happy with second place.

●●●●●●●●●●●●●●●●●●●●

WHOEVER SAID WINNING ISN'T EVERYTHING never had to explain to his wife how far ahead he was before losing his shirt in the Friday-night poker game. Nor could he have felt the joy of holding a softball trophy after years of distant finishes. Fact is, no matter how you play the game, winning beats the hell out of losing.

Keeping body and mind sharp can help put you on the winning side of most of life's little contests, but it's not always enough. Sometimes you need a bit of an edge, a strategy that the other guy doesn't know about. "Most times the difference between winning and losing is so small that all it takes to turn the tables is one little secret," says Mike Ray, the number one–ranked pro racquetball player in the country for three years running.

Over the past year, we've coaxed and cajoled trade secrets from experts in all types of competitive endeavors, from golf to fishing. Memorize what they have to say about your favorite contest, then hide this book from the friends you compete against. Let them be the ones consoling themselves with platitudes about how winning isn't everything.

GOLF

BRAD FAXON, EIGHTH-HIGHEST MONEY WINNER ON THE PROFESSIONAL GOLFERS' ASSOCIATION 1992 TOUR

1. Loosen your grip. Club head speed, which is what generates power, is unrelated to your strength, so a death grip isn't necessary. "Hold the club as if it were a tube of toothpaste," says Faxon.

2. Be a pessimist in club selection. Golfers tend to choose clubs based on their best performance with that club.

"Nine times out of ten they wind up hitting the ball short," says Faxon. Pick a club that's one size longer than you think you need.

3. Check your lie. Golf clubs take a terrific pounding and over time can be damaged. If the lie of a club is off, it can cause even the best-hit ball to veer off course. Have a golf shop check all your clubs at the beginning of each season.

TIC-TAC-TOE

PETER GORDON, ASSOCIATE EDITOR, *GAMES* MAGAZINE

1. Go first whenever possible. "A well-played game should always end in a tie," says Gordon. "But by going first you can ensure yourself the best odds of winning." Here's how you do it. Place your X in the center. If your opponent picks a noncorner square, you have the game won. Simply place your next X in one of the corners adjacent to your opponent. He'll be forced to block you. Then place your third X in the corner that will set you up for a two-way win that can't be blocked. If you start in the center and your opponent goes to a corner, there's not much you can do to win unless he makes a mistake. But the best strategy is to go for the corners and block when necessary.

2. If you must go second, try for a draw. Should your opponent start in the middle (and if he doesn't, he's a fool), put your first mark in a corner, then, as above, block wherever necessary. Should he *not* start in the middle square, place your O there and follow the initial strategy.

BASS FISHING

LARRY NIXON, ONLY FISHERMAN TO WIN MORE THAN $1 MILLION IN BASS-FISHING TOURNAMENTS

1. Fish the edges. Game fish such as bass, trout, crappie and walleye tend to hide out in weeds near the shoreline. Instead of casting your line as far as you can (a common beginner's mistake), try fishing from places where points of land jut out into the water. Keep moving if you're having no luck.

2. Think like a fish. In cloudy weather, bass usually feed off the surface, so top-water plugs or spinner baits work best. But on sunny days, bass move into the weeds and feed near the bottom, so plastic worms work then. "Plastic worms are the most efficient shoreline bait there is for bass fishing," says Nixon.

3. Use a deodorant. Many fish can detect a human smell on the lures. To conceal it, try spraying your lures with a fake scent. "I've had a lot of luck with crawfish scent," says Nixon.

MONOPOLY

LEE WEISENTHAL, FOUNDER, UNITED STATES MONOPOLY ASSOCIATION

1. Don't save money. As the game opens, buy everything you land on. "You can always mortgage or sell your properties if you need cash," says Weisenthal. Exceptions: utilities and railroads, which are not developable.

2. Get into the red and orange. Computer analysis has shown that the red and orange properties are the most landed on (a function of players being sent to jail and coming out on that side of the board). Make a special effort to buy and develop in this high-traffic area.

3. Wait to build. Don't start putting up houses until you can afford at least three. "The return on one or two houses is very small, but once you go to three, your investment starts to pay off," says Weisenthal. "It even pays to mortgage one of your other properties to build that third house."

RUNNING

JEFF GALLOWAY, AUTHOR, *GALLOWAY'S BOOK ON RUNNING;* MEMBER, 1972 U.S. OLYMPIC MARATHON TEAM

1. Go long. When preparing for a race, get out for a long run (one hour or longer) once a week to make your body more efficient at turning fat into fuel. To balance this long run and to prevent your muscles from getting injured, keep your other runs on the short side—say, three to six miles.

2. Get flats. If you plan on running a race that's less than ten kilometers (6.2 miles), try wearing running flats, which are ultralight racing shoes. "The weight difference between a heavy training shoe and a racing flat can save you several seconds a mile," says Galloway. One warning: If you weigh more than 180 pounds, flats won't give you enough support.

3. Lose weight. For every pound of fat you lose, you can shave two to five seconds off every mile.

NINTENDO

JEFFREY HANSEN, 13, 1991 WORLD NINTENDO CHAMPION

Be aggressive. In Nintendo as in life, you have to take chances if you want to win. "Fight everybody," says Hansen. This particularly holds true for winning at the popular Street Fighter II. Don't wait; run toward your opponent and hit him with everything you've got before he can pull any fancy moves.

CYCLING

LEN PETTYJOHN, DIRECTOR, COORS LITE CYCLING TEAM

1. Ride in low gears. Although pushing a high gear can make you go faster, it will also tire you more quickly. To go faster longer, use a gear low enough to turn the pedals at least 70 times per minute.

2. Connect to your pedals. Bike pedals with straps to hold your feet allow you to pull up on one pedal while pushing down on the other. This added force can increase your speed by one to two miles per hour. Also, get proper stiff-soled biking shoes, which allow you to apply more pressure to the pedals. "Soft, flexible running shoes are the worst things to ride in," says Pettyjohn.

3. Lighten up. The lighter your wheels, the easier it will be to get them moving. Sometimes the change can be as easy as having your bike shop switch you to lighter spokes, but it may also be necessary to use a lighter rim or hub.

CHESS

DAN EDELMAN, ASSOCIATE DIRECTOR, U.S. CHESS FEDERATION

1. Have a good opening line. Getting a chess book and learning several openings will help you to establish a good setup early in the game. "Many times the whole tone of a chess game is set in the first ten moves," says Edelman.

2. Control the center. The four squares in the center of the board are the most important, since they allow quick access to all four quadrants. Do what you can to gain control of this area as soon as possible.

3. Trade up. When you're behind, trade only to take a piece of higher value; when you're ahead, it's to your advantage to trade pieces of equal value.

4. Castle early. Obviously, the name of the game is to protect your king. Castling quickly and efficiently tucks him out of harm's way.

RACQUETBALL

MIKE RAY, TOP-RANKED U.S. PROFESSIONAL RACQUETBALL PLAYER

1. Think big. Buy the biggest, lightest racket you can find. Wide-body frames give you more reach and also allow you to hit the ball 20 to 30 miles per hour faster than a conventional racket.

2. Run them off the court. "Players tend to practice hitting the ball while standing still," says Ray. "Keep them moving, and chances are you'll throw them off their game." You'll also wear them out.

3. Wear a glove. A glove gives you a better grip on the racket. As a general rule, get one that's a size smaller than your normal glove. (A loose-fitting glove will allow the racket to slip in your hand.)

4. Scrape your shoes. The urethane on the soles of new shoes can cause you to lose traction on the court. Always scuff the bottoms of your shoes on macadam before playing in them.

ARM WRESTLING

WAYNE BURNS, 1991 WORLD ARM-WRESTLING CHAMPION IN THE 65-KILOGRAM DIVISION

1. Grip high. By getting a high grip on your opponent's thumb, you automatically increase your leverage and your chances of winning.

2. Stay close. Always keep the distance between your hand and body as short as possible, because the closer you are, the more leverage you get.

3. Start fast. Most arm-wrestling matches are over in under ten seconds, and usually the one who makes the first strong move wins. "Hit hard and keep pulling," says Burns.

VOLLEYBALL

BRYAN IVIE, STARTING MIDDLE BLOCKER, BRONZE-MEDAL 1992 U.S. OLYMPIC VOLLEYBALL TEAM

1. Take your eye off the ball. Instead, key on your opponent's torso and shoulders, and position yourself accordingly. "When you're blocking a shot, if you're watching only the ball, it'll be by you before you have time to react," suggests Ivie.

2. Feet first. One of the most common mistakes volleyball players make when going for a ball is to reach with their arms. Instead, first move your feet and position yourself squarely behind the ball.

3. Wear the right shoes. Basketball shoes, commonly worn by novice players, are much heavier than volleyball shoes, and the extra weight can cut into your jump and slow you down.

FOOTBALL POOLS

NORM HITZGES, ESPN PROGNOSTICATOR

1. Always take the road underdog getting 1 to 2.5 points. The average fan realizes that the home team has an advantage, so when they see a close game, they'll usually take the home team and give the points. But oddsmakers build in a 3-point advantage for the home team. So a spread of less than 3 points means the road team is actually stronger than the home team. "I'd take a better team over the home-field advantage anytime, especially when they're getting points," says Hitzges.

2. Take the underdog when getting 6 points, and take the favorite when laying 7 to 14 points. The 6- to 6.5-point spread is designed to get people thinking all they need is a touchdown to cover the spread. But in reality the favorite may not be significantly better than the underdog. On the other hand, any team that oddsmakers favor by more than a touchdown has to be far better than the other team.

3. Pick the stronger league. Recently, the NFC has been much stronger than the AFC, so when in doubt on a close call, go for the NFC team.

TENNIS

VIC BRADEN, TEACHING PRO FOR 40 YEARS; FOUNDER AND PRESIDENT OF THE VIC BRADEN TENNIS COLLEGE

1. Hit one extra ball. In a typical rally, a tennis player will attempt to put away the ball on his third shot. But for the average player, attempting a putaway is risky business. "Studies have shown that being patient and hitting back one more ball than you normally do will allow you to beat over 50 percent of the people who now beat you," says Braden.

2. Keep your head down. Concentrate on watching the ball hit your racket. "Your brain works one-fifth of a second ahead of your muscles, so by the time you're about to hit the ball, your brain is already thinking about your next shot," says Braden. This delay causes many players to lift their heads before they actually hit the ball.

3. When in doubt, hit crosscourt. You're less likely to hit a ball out of bounds or into the net if you hit the ball on a diagonal.

DARTS

TOM FLEETWOOD, COFOUNDER AND EXECUTIVE DIRECTOR, AMERICAN DARTS ORGANIZATION

1. Loosen your grip. Hold your dart as you would hold a small bird.

2. Keep both eyes open. Closing one eye will throw off your depth perception.

3. Push, don't throw. Start with the dart at the side of your head just in front of your eye; then moving only your elbow, push it toward the board. Never pull the dart back behind your field of vision. "You should be able to see the dart at all times," says Fleetwood.

SWIMMING

NORT THORNTON, COACH OF MATT BIONDI (NINE-TIME GOLD MEDAL WINNER FOR THE U.S. OLYMPIC SWIM TEAM); MEN'S SWIMMING COACH AT THE UNIVERSITY OF CALIFORNIA, BERKELEY

1. Concentrate on your center. "Many swimmers focus on their extremities to generate power, but the most power comes from your hips," says Thornton. When swimming freestyle, your hips should turn perpendicular to the water.

2. Accentuate your out-breath. To take in more air, forcefully exhale before lifting your head to breathe. This creates a strong suction and brings in more air. "Many swimmers use only about 10 percent of their lung capacity," says Thornton.

POKER

STEVE FOX, EXECUTIVE DIRECTOR, NATIONAL POKER ASSOCIATION

1. Never chase a hand. Fold a seven card stud hand if you don't start with at least a pair, three cards of the same suit or the middle three cards of a straight. Fold a draw poker hand if you don't have a pair of jacks or better. "Good poker players win fewer hands but take home more money," says Fox, who frequently comes out ahead by winning as few as *two* hands in an evening.

2. Choose your game wisely. Dealer's choice? Pick five card draw, no wild cards. Five card draw always gives the dealer an advantage, since he gets to go last after he's had a chance to gauge the strength of his opponents' hands by their discards and bets. The reason to stay away from wild cards is that they can obliterate the dealer's advantage by too easily changing a weak hand to a strong one.

3. Don't sort your cards. When playing draw poker, a clever opponent will spot your sorting habits and deduce what type of hand you've been dealt. When playing stud games, look at your down cards only when they're dealt to you. Checking them again gives opponents valuable information about your hand. Say it's seven card stud and you have a pair of aces down and a nine of spades up. Your next up card is jack of spades. If you check to see if one of your aces is a spade, this reveals that you probably have a pair down, that the pair *aren't* jacks and that now you might be thinking about a flush.

SOFTBALL

BRUCE MEADE, U.S. SLO-PITCH SOFTBALL ASSOCIATION HALL-OF-FAMER

1. Don't hit up on the ball. Swinging up is likely to produce more pop flies than hits. "Swing level and look for gaps between players," says Meade.

2. Hit short pitches. In slo-pitch, the best pitches to swing through are those that come down in front of you, giving you a chance to step into the ball.

3. Stay loose. Keep your arms and shoulders relaxed when at the plate. Tensing up and trying to overmuscle the ball will throw off your swing.

4. Go for metal. "Using an aluminum bat will give you 50 more feet of hitting power than a wooden bat," says Meade.

BOWLING

DICK WEBER, PROFESSIONAL BOWLERS ASSOCIATION HALL-OF-FAMER

1. Don't twist. Many bowlers bring their arms across their bodies or turn their wrists as they release the ball, which throws them off balance. Your shoulders should be parallel with the foul line, and your throwing arm should follow a pendulum path at your side.

2. Don't overpower the pins. Throwing the ball too hard can cause the pins to fly around too much and miss each other. "A well-thrown ball at medium speed lays the pins down flatter and allows them to mix," explains Weber.

FLAG FOOTBALL

BRIAN BROOMELL, QUARTERBACK, 1991 NATIONAL FLAG FOOTBALL CHAMPIONSHIP TEAM

1. Throw short. Because flag football is usually played without the two tackles, quarterbacks have a smaller pocket and less time to throw deep. "Short posts, slants and crossing patterns under ten yards are easy to complete and keep the offense's momentum high," says Broomell.

2. Practice grabbing flags. Although it may look easy, ripping a flag off a fullback who's moving downfield with a full head of steam can be quite a task. So during practice, spend 10 or 15 minutes simply working on grabbing your teammates' flags.

POOL

MIKE FUSCO, PROFESSIONAL POOL PLAYER AND PROTÉGÉ OF POOL GREAT WILLIE MOSCONI

1. Stay down. Many beginning players lean over while aiming their shot and then stand before they're finished. For the greatest accuracy, stay down until you completely finish your follow-through.

2. Chalk it up. Do it after every shot. A well-chalked stick is less likely to slip off the cue ball and cause you to miss your shot.

3. Easy does it. Go for an easy, smooth shot with a good follow-through. If you hit the cue ball hard, it will actually leave the table for a split second and change direction.

CHECKERS

CHARLES C. WALKER, DIRECTOR, INTERNATIONAL CHECKER HALL OF FAME

1. Move to the middle. By moving your pieces toward the center rather than the edges, you double your options.

2. Keep it together. Before offering a piece to your opponent, make sure you have at least two other pieces stacked behind it. "This will keep you from getting burned with a double or triple jump," says Walker.

3. Run to the corner. If you're down a king at the end, it pays to hide out in a corner and move back and forth there. "It takes some skill to get someone out of a corner, and the average player usually loses a piece or two in the process," says Walker. If your opponent does roust you out of the corner, run for the opposite one.

SKEET SHOOTING

WAYNE MAYES, 28-TIME WORLD SKEET-SHOOTING CHAMPION

1. Stay with the gun. The most common problem skeet shooters have is taking the gun off their shoulder too quickly. That breaks the gun's momentum and wastes the tail end of the shot. "Stay with the target after you pull the trigger," Mayes recommends.

2. Use both eyes. Although closing one eye may make it easier to aim the gun at first, doing so will throw off your depth perception and interfere with your peripheral vision. From the very beginning, it's best to get used to shooting with both eyes open. "All the best skeet shooters use both eyes," says Mayes.

3. And get them both checked. In the course of a year, it's possible for your vision to change enough to throw off your shot. To keep your shooting at its best, have your eyes checked at the beginning of every year.

PINBALL

DOUG YOUNG, EXECUTIVE DIRECTOR, INTERNATIONAL FLIPPER PINBALL ASSOCIATION

Read the directions. All pinball games have a set of directions on the top glass next to the left flipper. Reading them will tell you which targets you need to hit and in what order to score the most points. "Just smashing the ball around for five minutes will get you some points, but don't expect high scores that way," says Young.

—*Dan Bensimhon*

Part 4

MAN-TO-MAN TALK

Talking Money

*Why is it that a man can easily discuss
his prostate, his mistress, his bald spot,
almost anything—yet squirms when the subject
is money?*

• • • • • • • • • • • • • • • • • • •

I HAVE A FRIEND—we all have this friend, in one guise or another—who once lived a life of sublime simplicity: small house, small bed, small bills. He was a happy man with only one failing: He didn't know how to talk money.

How he came to realize this shortcoming is a lesson to us all. He met a beautiful woman with a big wardrobe and three children, and he married her. He needed a larger home, of course, so he bought one. The kids needed braces; the wife needed cars. The complications of his life soon formed a mountain of paper—invoices, demands, threats—on his desk. He wasn't sleeping well, so he moved to the couch at night. This eventually angered his wife, who moved in with the guy who cleaned the pool, leaving my friend with the charming children and a bed all to himself. The children soon became adolescents, and one of them was arrested. To make bail, the guy had to take out a lien on the house. It became impossible to pay alimony, so the court started hounding him. He lost the house and moved into an apartment. This embarrassed the kids, who began to have more problems. One thing led to another, until finally his boss called him on the carpet and asked why he was missing work, why the courthouse was calling the personnel office and why he was so damned irritable. The guy certainly knew what was wrong: He'd hit the black ice of poverty and skidded out of control. He was broke and getting more broke. But it was all too embarrassing. Since he didn't know what to say, he skipped all the symptoms and went straight for the cure: He demanded a raise. His boss fired him.

Now the pitiable subject of our little lecture may have been forgiven for his inability to discuss money once. After all, when he met the woman who became the instrument of his undoing, he should have simply asked "Nice, but how much?" Maybe he didn't want to look at lust with jaded eyes. Or maybe he was just worried that he couldn't afford the woman and the excess baggage of her life. Whichever, he signed on and paid the price in long, painful installments.

But it was only shortly after the wedding that he became desperate for money. Money invaded his every thought. His boss, an affable fellow, was the one man who had the ability to deliver our man from bondage. Long before he was fired, I asked him why he didn't go to his boss and try to work something out. "I could never do that," he said. "I hate talking money with people."

So he never did—until it came time to come clean. Then he started talking money when he should have been talking contrition.

LESSON TO BE LEARNED

So our lesson will be found in the answer to this mild, commonplace question: Why can a man talk prostate, talk infidelity, talk atrocity and theft, yet still not be able to talk turkey?

First off, men do not understand what money is for. This is why women are better at asking for, and receiving, raises than men are. For many men, money is God's yardstick. It is the immutable measure, the absolute dimension of a man's worth, and to talk about it is to open a discussion about lots of important things, such as power, self-esteem, conflict, humiliation and generosity. Women have lives considerably more complex than most men's, so they tend to see money much more clearly. To a normal woman, money isn't some compli-

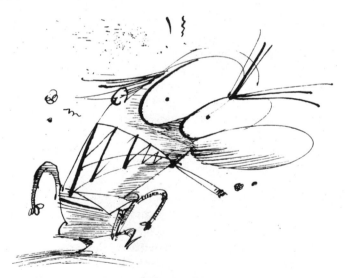

Hostile Habits

If you're a hostile guy, chances are you have some unhealthy habits. In a 2½-year study, scientists found that men who scored high on a test of hostility tended to have high intakes of cholesterol and sugar and low intakes of calcium. These cranky men also tended to smoke more than their easy-going counterparts. On the plus side, the hostile subjects tended to get more exercise and have lower systolic blood pressure.

cated scoring device in the full-body contact sport of life. To women, money is what you use to buy stuff.

This is not to say women object to men making lots of money. In fact, many women *love* men who make lots of money. Back in the 1960s and 1970s, would-be rock stars used to stuff a sock in their pants to make a mighty love muscle. But maybe they missed the point, because some women weren't looking at love Lugers so much as they were checking out the *other* bulge—the money bulge, the one a wallet makes, the one that counts.

Because men confuse money with every other estimable virtue—intelligence, muscle, power, whatever—money is a volatile subject. When money's the topic between two men, conflict is in the air. The guy who has the money hates the other guy for trying to get some of it. The guy who wants the money hates the other guy for making him ask for it—it should be offered to him, he figures, because it's so obvious that he's skilled, or talented, or a nice guy, or a brother-in-law. Consequently, men who dislike confrontation can never discuss money. Instead, they stew about it in silence.

So how do you talk money? First, you have to get comfortable with the stuff. Try these relaxation techniques.

Demystify it. A pile of money sitting in a room with nobody around has no mojo. To paraphrase writer P. J. O'Rourke, you can't smoke it, you can't eat it, you can't f— it, so what good is it? Look at a sawbuck closely. Meditate on it. Get to know it. Think difficult thoughts. Why should it take *20* George Washingtons to make one lousy Andy Jackson? How does this impact your life?

Don't measure yourself with it. Remember, a dollar bill is only six inches long, and six inches isn't much.

Do something stupid with it. Demonstrate its worthlessness to yourself. Buy a snowmobile. Feed it to goats. Or overtip your way into the life of a cocktail waitress.

Next, recognize what kind of money you're talking about. There are two kinds of money: yours and theirs. For example, to you, your money is American money. You comprehend its worth almost intuitively. It has a familiar feel, a comfortable texture. A stack of it has an overupholstered exuberance that, when placed in your pocket in a thick roll, puts a spring in your step and a smile on your face. A huge, fat wad of bills in your hand is what immortality feels like.

Their money is foreign currency. When somebody starts talking to you about money that isn't your own (even though, perhaps, it ought to be), it's as if they were quoting hog-belly futures in zlotys. You can't possibly understand the worth of somebody else's money because you don't know how much of it they *have*. If Mother Teresa gave you a C-note, it would seem like a fortune. If Howard Hughes gave you the same hundred-dollar bill, you'd think it was chump change.

THE LAW OF MONEY MIGRATION

All you can know for sure about *their* money is that it exerts a gravitational pull on you. There is physics involved here, actually, and the rule goes like this: The strength of the gravitational pull from somebody else's bankroll is directly proportional to the degree of your conviction that it rightly belongs to you.

For example, let's say you walk into the boss's office looking for a bonus. You know what you've done to earn it, and so does he. You have a dollar figure in mind, and so does he. (And believe it or not, these two figures will be phenomenally close almost every time.)

You can feel the tug of his money; it's like a bass at the end of a line. His job is to get that money of his to behave and stop trying to wiggle out of his pocket and into yours. Your job is to stand up for your conviction that you are offering that money its rightful place.

Ultimately, of course, when you're talking money, you're talking power, and power is the big Harley of life, the one that rides you unless you learn to ride it. Power is best seen as something God doles out to a lucky few just to impose a little order on an uncivilized world. If you have power, the best advice is to play the benevolent despot—firm but caring and, above all, fair—since what you do with power is a better measure of your worth than the half-foot of a dollar bill. And if you are a petitioner, make fairness your own talking point, since no deal is a good deal unless it's a good deal on both sides. But above all, as my friend learned too late, remember that if you're going to talk money, make sure money's the topic of conversation.

—Denis Boyles

Mastering Fear

Go on the Fear Diet. You'll shed your
anxiety like so many unwanted pounds.
Satisfaction guaranteed ... or your panic back.

● ● ● ● ● ● ● ● ● ● ● ● ● ● ● ● ● ● ●

> Courage is resistance to fear, mastery of fear—not
> absence of fear.
>
> *—Mark Twain*

IT'S EVERYWHERE, LIKE a deadly, contagious virus. It's
fear, especially fear of economic insecurity. A close friend
calls and says that he has only one month's mortgage payment in the bank—that if he loses his job, he would lose his
home. Another calls to say her business may have to close.
She's an engineer, and if she loses her job in Los Angeles at
this moment, she will have an incredibly hard time getting
another one like it. On TV, there are scenes of the largest
employer in the San Fernando Valley, a huge auto plant,
closing down. Thousands will lose their jobs, and there are
no likely replacements on the scene.

Fear. I have it in my life, too. I have three mortgages to
pay—taken out in far balmier days for both me and the real-
estate market—an extremely expensive assistant, insurance
bills that will not quit and the need to provide for retirement
some 20 years down the road, all out of a livelihood that is
steadily more dicey in a steadily worse economy.

Occasionally, I wake up from this fear at 5:00 in the
morning, sometimes with a crushing pain in my chest and
sweats starting out in my toes and reaching up to my scalp.

When this happens, I take a number of mental and
physical steps. In my mind, I have come to refer to them as
the Fear Diet. It's a plan of thinking and living that has
helped me—and that I hope will continue to help me—lose
fear, little by little, ounce by ounce, until I am no longer
bloated with it and can handle my daily life—even the part at
5:00 A.M.—without that crushing burden.

GET UP

First, I get up and get out of bed. There is no more vulnerable place to be when panic strikes than in bed, under the covers, prone. I get up and get the paper, turn on the morning TV shows and see that life goes on.

I get dressed and go outside and see that there are cars and people and trees and birds and that life continues to push up flowers from under the ground. It puts my terror into a certain perspective and makes it small.

GO WITH THE FLOW

Second, I exercise. Not very much, to be sure, but enough to get the blood flowing. I do sit ups and push ups and lift weights and walk my dog a few blocks up and down steep hills. This truly works wonders. There's a chemical basis for fear, something about secretions of hormones. Exercise alters that function, replaces the fear chemical with a getting-by one, prepares me to believe I can at least get through until lunch, which is no small thing when I am afraid that the next homeless man is going to be me.

CHANT FOR COURAGE

Third, I sing. That's right, I sing. In particular, I sing a famous song of the civil rights movement called "We Shall Overcome." The lines I particularly love to sing, while walking early in the morning with my dog, go something like this.

We are not afraid,
We are not afraid,
We are not afraid today.
Oh, deep in my heart, I do believe,
We are not afraid today.

You may laugh at this, and I probably would have before I saw brave men and women singing it while getting bitten by police dogs and knocked down by fire hoses in Birmingham in 1964 and keeping their courage—in part, I like to think, because they came to believe what they sang.

If you don't know the tune, get it from someone middle-aged who worked in the civil rights movement. It's a great song, and it can turn a day of fear of the bank into a day of achievement.

● ●

SAY IT AIN'T SO

Panic can strike anytime: not just in bed in the middle of the night but at work, in the shower before work, in the deli at lunchtime, in the car on the way home. Emmett Miller, M.D., medical director of the Cancer Support and Education Center in Menlo Park, California, and a nationally known expert on stress, offers these suggestions.

SET PRIORITIES

The following phrases can help you unwind when unpleasant thoughts knot the muscles in your neck and tension mounts.

- "There's no place I have to go at this moment in time."
- "There's no problem I have to solve at this moment in time."
- "There's nothing I have to do at this moment in time."
- "The most important thing I can experience at this moment in time is relaxation."

It's necessary to think these thoughts consciously, Dr. Miller says, because doing so automatically changes the mindset that's producing the stress. If you're reciting the litany, you're not thinking about whatever bothers you.

THINK POSITIVE

Reviewing a past success, particularly before a presentation or a meeting with your boss, is an excellent way to eradicate the butterflies: "You're instantly reminded that you've achieved before, and there's no reason you shouldn't achieve this time," says Dr. Miller.

"You should have a list of affirmations ready that you can start repeating when you feel stressed," Dr. Miller says. "They don't have to be complicated. Just thinking to yourself 'I can handle this' or 'I know more about this than anyone here' will work. It pulls you away from the animal reflex to stress—the quick breathing, the cold hands—and toward the reasoned response, the intellect—the part of you that really can handle it."

The result? You calm down.

● ●

FOOD VS. FEAR

Fourth, I eat something simple. Usually, it's toast and orange juice, the basic foods of the morning and of decades of familiarity. It's hard to be afraid when I'm eating, and it's especially hard to be in fear when the sugar and other nutrients from whatever I eat are entering my bloodstream. It's not just coincidence that people in fear like to eat. Metabolized food is energizing, refreshing, calming. (There's an obvious problem here in terms of possible excess, but that's another story.)

TALK TO MYSELF

Fifth, I sit down to my work, and as I do, I tell myself some extremely basic facts about fear, life and me.

■ When I am in fear of the future, I try to imagine the worst that could possibly happen—that I would lose my house. So what? I had my happiest moments when I was living in a one-room apartment in the middle of nowhere. Lose my fancy car? I was happier when I had a ten-year-old clunker. If the worst happens, I'll still have a roof, Mozart tapes and decent food, and that's not bad.

■ When I am in fear over what I do not have now, especially things such as money, property and prestige, I think about what I do have: a wonderful five-year-old son, a great dog, a devoted former wife, more friends than anyone else I know, interesting work and a brilliant, still-lively set of parents. The list goes on and on, and every entry wipes away a lot of fear.

■ When I am in fear that paralyzes me, I try to act like an economist of my own life. I remind myself that there is no value-added in fear, that there is no profit in fear, that there is no pleasure in fear, that there is no wisdom in fear.

■ When I feel ashamed for having money problems, I realize that I am far from being alone in them. I didn't commit any crimes by buying real estate when everyone thought it was a great idea. If the biggest banks and the most astute real-estate developers in the world made the same mistake, I can hardly blame myself for making it.

■ When I am in fear that my life is wasted, I make a list of every good thing I have ever done, and then I allow myself to feel proud about them. I busted a financial fraud in one place. I saved a lot of homeless animals in another. I got up in the morning and played with my son even though I was exhausted. Above all, I forgave a number of people who had been truly vicious to me. So by comparison, the mistakes I have made seem smaller than the things I've done right.

▪ No matter what, as I lie in bed or get to my desk and have fear wash over me, I am not going to let the recession or the real-estate collapse or any other thing make me angry toward my son or make me commit violence against myself by a heart attack or in any other way. I have no power over the economy, but I do have power over me, and I am going to use it to make my life better, not end it.

▪ Oh, and one other thing: I get plenty of rest. It's almost impossible to feel secure when you're exhausted or frightened.

That's it. Try it. If it doesn't work, you can always have your fear back, guaranteed.

—*Benjamin Stein*

Releasing Control

Needing control when we can't have it is a decidely unhealthy, even deadly, mix. Here's how to break free of this common male trap.

• • • • • • • • • • • • • • • • • •

ASK ME TO DESCRIBE A ROUTINE source of personal stress, and I'll be very precise: a Harley-Davidson, no apparent muffler, ridden by a fat guy with a scraggly beard, black jeans, a leather vest and an attitude. I have in mind not a particular guy but rather a legion of them that roars regularly past my house, an architectural gem situated on the corner of a busy urban neighborhood. It's a fine place to live, but the street outside seems to be a main route for outlaw bikers to get wherever it is that outlaw bikers go. Now I have nothing against motorcycles. However, when the explosive din from their pistons drowns out a normal conversation in my own living room, it drives me crazy. The problem is, aside from packing up my family and moving to some remote corner of the earth, there's not a thing I can do about it. Instead, whenever a loud bike snarls past, I fantasize about the damage I could do to it with a baseball bat, or I mentally replay the concluding scenes of *Easy Rider,* secretly and shamefully cheering the redneck farmer who blows Dennis Hopper and Peter Fonda off their mounts with a shotgun. Not that I make a big show of my feelings. I take a deep breath. I clench my teeth. I slowly shake my head. My wife, on the other hand, recognizing all the signs of my inner seething, gently admonishes me to calm down. The noise doesn't seem to faze her in the least.

Ask any man to tell you about the stress in his life, and the key issue is likely to be the same as it is for me: lack of control. "This is one of the greatest stresses men have," says psychiatrist David Baron, D.O., medical director of the Horsham Clinic, outside Philadelphia. "Control issues are frequently more important for men than they are for women."

That's because women don't share our Mr. Fixit mentality. They tend to see the big picture, to ask what real harm is being done and to put top priority on how a stressful event affects the relationships in their lives. "Women have very effective coping mechanisms in talking with friends and allowing themselves to have a good cry when life gets overwhelming, but men aren't taught to do that stuff," says Kenneth Wetcher, M.D., a Houston-based psychiatrist who specializes in men's issues.

The control principle holds true for stresses large and small alike. Why do we men go crazy in traffic jams and supermarket lines? Why do we prefer being behind the wheel to being a passenger? Why do we detest going to a doctor or dentist? Why do we avoid asking directions when we're lost? Why do we love winning? Why do we hate being sick or the thought of getting old? "Control, control, control," as Steve Martin intones to Kevin Kline at the start of the movie *Grand Canyon.*

SORRY, YOU CAN'T HAVE IT

There's just one problem with control: We often can't have it. "When are you going to realize that nothing can be controlled?" Martin continues in his harangue to Kline. Minutes later, Kline becomes lost in a dangerous L.A. neighborhood, his car breaks down, he's menaced by thugs, and he is saved only by happenstance.

"Things happen, and the less control you feel, the more you want to have it, which makes you feel even more out of control," says Herbert J. Freudenberger, Ph.D., an authority on burnout. "It becomes a vicious cycle that only makes stress worse."

This cycle is especially vicious to men because our physical response to stress is different from women's. For one thing, our blood pressure tends to shoot higher when we're under stress, which, over time, puts us at greater risk of heart disease and stroke, diseases that fell 25- to 64-year-old men 2.4 times more than women.

What's the deal with men and control? Why is it so important to us? According to one view, it stems partly from evolutionary urges hard-wired into our genes. Consider what the stress response really is: a fight-or-flight instinct that we developed back when we spent a lot of time in close company with wild and hungry beasts. In those days, "control" meant action, not just to defend yourself but also to protect your entire family. Failing to take action meant you and your loved ones were dead.

The main reason men like to keep a firm grip on the control stick, however, is that we're *taught* to. Control is necessary if you're to be what a man in our culture is supposed to be: strong, self-reliant, successful and all-knowing. The standard male hero has control in spades. With Humphrey Bogart, to cite a personal favorite, there's no real suspense about whether he'll come out on top, because you know he always will and he acts like *he* knows it. He's impressive precisely because he maintains steely control even when the other guys have the drop on him.

"When we're in control, we feel like victors and successes," says Dr. Baron, "and when we're out of control, every little thing becomes stressful."

NOT THE SAME FOR WOMEN

It just isn't the same for women. One important reason is that the prospect of motherhood leads women to expect a certain lack of control during life. Furthermore, women are raised to live up to a different set of standards, most of which revolve around the less control-oriented issues of family and relationships. "Girls are raised to be 'good,' " says psychologist Georgia Witkin-Lanoil, Ph.D., author of *The Female*

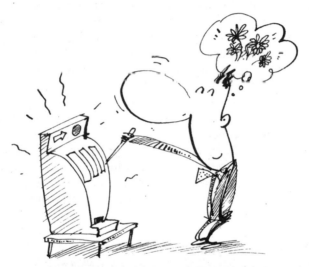

Pay through the Nose

Gambling casinos are sensual palaces designed to put you in the mood to spend money: soft lights, plush carpets, scantily clad waitresses. Someday casinos may have another trick up their sleeves: scents that make you want to play until you are down to the lint in your pockets. When Alan R. Hirsch, M.D., neurologic director of the Smell and Taste Treatment and Research Foundation in Chicago, released an appealing scent through a row of slot machines at a Las Vegas casino over a weekend, gamblers blew an average of 45 percent more cash. Although Dr. Hirsch won't reveal the aroma (it's a trade secret, he says), he explains that certain fragrances trigger nostalgic, even childlike, emotions in people, who may then be more willing to feed a slot machine.

Stress Syndrome. "They are praised and rewarded when they are empathetic, conforming and considerate." Pressured to be pictures of perfection, they're most stressed by situations where they feel they'll let people down.

On the home front, the male need for control is often rooted in something deeper: responsibility. We learn early on that being a man means being responsible for everyone's overall security and comfort. This isn't a bad thing. Psychologists point to our traditional commitment to our families and our setting aside of our own needs for those of our loved ones as some of the best qualities men possess.

But responsibility to always be the provider can take its toll. Good providers, after all, must know how to fix *any* problem that pops up, from leaky faucets to cracks in the driveway to a child's falling math scores to the federal deficit. And good providers must have a steady income, even if that means sacrificing personal goals. "Unlike women, many men don't feel they have any choice in this matter," says Dr. Baron. Being a responsible provider "is a persistent, chronic source of stress that men have to deal with every day, and it's a big reason why a man's career success may have a greater bearing on his self-esteem and mental health than anything else."

THE ROAD TO BURNOUT

For some of us, the provider ethic translates into a drive to make lots of money. For others, it becomes a compulsion to outperform everyone around us. By being the better worker, we become the better man. When the boss suggests we take on another project, we don't want to let on that we're overwhelmed, and we don't know how to say no. "That's when you find yourself working nights and weekends," Dr. Freudenberger says. And heading down the road to burnout.

These tendencies are particularly strong in men who have hard-driving, aggressive Type A personalities, the hallmarks of which are found almost exclusively in men. In fact, just about every man has a little Type A in him, according to C. David Jenkins, Ph.D., professor of preventive medicine and community health at the University of Texas Medical Branch at Galveston. Type A men often struggle with a relentless urge to maintain control and flare into a rage when they can't.

Another problem zone is relationships with women. Because women respond to stress in different ways than men do, simple arguments can seem like border disputes between countries with different languages. When the pressure's on, for us the need to be problem solvers is paramount. Because of this, trying to talk about disagreements is messy. We'd prefer to figure out problems on our own, without asking for help or bringing her into it. Women don't need solutions as quickly. They're satisfied to talk out their problems, and they often try to get us to do the same.

The result is that we often don't bring up problems or annoyances until we're so bugged by them that we can't hold them in any longer. Then we come across as hostile, and the result is an explosion. The more solution-oriented you are, the tougher your relationships will be, experts say, because you'll be less flexible and less willing to see your partner's point of view. Such rigidity may not have mattered in the man's-home-is-his-castle days, but it puts you at a definite disadvantage in the era of dual-income households, when everything from chores to career decisions is open to negotiation. "If you argue about every little thing, she'll be less likely to compromise on issues that are important to you," Dr. Jenkins says.

THE PARADOX OF CONTROL

The paradox of control is that to feel like you have more of it, you need to loosen up on the reins. "If you let go of your need for control, you ease your stress," says Alvin Baraff, Ph.D., director of MenCenter in Washington, D.C. "Letting go is a way of giving yourself options."

In order to successfully let go—as distinguished from throwing in the towel—you need to invest in what Allen Elkin, Ph.D., program director of the Stress Management and Counseling Center in New York City, calls counter-control measures.

Be realistic. There's no harm in trying to improve a situation if taking action will really help. If you're having problems managing your workload, for example, look at whether

you could delegate responsibilities better or get more training. Instead of automatically saying yes to new tasks, tell
your boss you'll need to prioritize what's already on your
plate, and ask what jobs *he* thinks you should do first. If
you're facing a problem in a relationship, let your mate in on
your thinking. Ask what *she* thinks should be done. "Try it as
an experiment," says Dr. Baraff. "See if it isn't easier, if you
don't feel lighter and if you don't reach a solution faster."

Get some perspective. Step back from the problem to
keep yourself from overreacting. Next time you feel worked
up, rate what's stressing you on a scale of 0 to 10, suggests
Dr. Elkin. Then rate your reaction to it from 0 to 10 as well.
"Having trouble finding a parking space rates maybe a 1,"
Dr. Elkin says. "But if you're feeling more like 9, then you're
out of balance and need to lighten up a little."

Other perspective lenders: Ask yourself if you'll remember in three weeks what's bothering you today. If your
answer is no, your problem is probably not very important.
Try not to think about how things should or shouldn't be:
"This traffic system should have been designed better" or "I
shouldn't have to put up with this." *Shoulds* are beyond your
control. Focus instead on what *is*.

Look beneath the surface. Loosening the reins

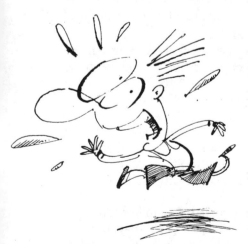

Healthy Sweat

If you tend to sweat more
than most people, it may be
because you're more physically fit than they are. A study
published in the *Physician
and Sportsmedicine* suggests
that physically active people
develop larger and more efficient sweat glands than people who are less fit. Their
glands, say the researchers,
respond to exercise in much
the same way muscles do:
They get bigger.

begins with values, Dr. Elkin says. "The common wisdom that nobody on his deathbed wishes he'd spent more time at the office may be trite, but it's true. We need to step back out of the jungle and ask what's really important in life."

One way of doing this is to challenge some of the assumptions that make control such a peculiarly male issue. In particular, Dr. Elkin advises looking at the standards by which you rate other people, because those will also be the standards by which you rate yourself. Do you tend to judge people based on their job title or the amount of money they make? Do you admire only the skillful? "Jim Courier plays better tennis than I do, but does that make him a better person? Of course not," Dr. Elkin says. "We're too complicated to be rated or judged by any measure other than who we are. Although we may like it, no man truly needs other people's approval."

Give something back. Look for ways to commit yourself to ideals beyond yourself. One review of more than 60 studies of stress-busting tactics found that having a sense of purpose in life was the single most powerful way for men to gain peace of mind. It may come from religious involvement in a church or synagogue, where a basic tenet is that control ultimately lies not with you but with a higher power. It may come from working for political reform or acting as a mentor for young people through activities such as Little League or Boy Scouts. It may even come from something as simple as a hobby or an intellectual pursuit that has nothing to do with your job.

Set goals for yourself. Having goals also helps channel the need for control beyond the day-to-day. Goals give us direction and provide a context for our travails. If your objective is to start your own business, even a lousy job becomes more bearable if it's providing experience you'll find useful later. If things don't work out the way you planned, take that as an opportunity to make new goals. The bottom line is to step back a bit from yourself and realize that controlling your problems won't necessarily solve them.

In all this, there are specific lessons for me to apply the next time a Harley-Davidson gets me hot under the collar. First, it's just not that big a deal. Second, it has no bearing on anything I truly hold dear. And third, the fact that it's beyond

my control is something to accept, not to fight mental battles
about. These are simple truths, but they help. I'm reminded
of how people responded to pressure back in the more laid-
back and less urban neighborhood that I grew up in. There,
when people were irked by something beyond their control,
they gave a shrug, looked toward the heavens and said simply, "What can you do?"

—*Richard Laliberte*

Men's Times

*A man may not know where he's going,
but he should always know where he's been.*

● ● ● ● ● ● ● ● ● ● ● ● ● ● ● ● ● ● ●

ALTHOUGH IT HAPPENED before my fourth birthday, I'll
never forget the afternoon I summoned enough courage to
pee in the big toilet—standing up, firing a sure stream into
the intimidating abyss like a man. It was a threshold
moment. But in the nearsighted thrill of victory, I failed to
see how this simple feat of bravery and skill would become a
milestone. I didn't know it at the time, but peeing in the toilet
was the culmination of my young life's work. It took years of
progression and coaching—from diapers through potty chair
to bowl-side practice sessions with Dad ("Hold it with two
fingers and watch what you're doing")—to reach the glorious moment when I could stand and deliver with some
degree of accuracy. This rite of passage forever separated
me from the ways of Mom and my sisters and put me on
equal footing, so to speak, with Dad and other standing
members of our male pee-er group.

Okay, 30 years later, standing up to pee for the first time
doesn't seem like such a big deal. But it happened, and it
changed the way I did something for the rest of my life. That
makes it a milestone. There are many such milestones in a

man's life. Some are more profound than others, and some are more predictable—birth, puberty and death, for instance.

Some milestones are biological, such as sprouting your first scraggly facial hairs. Others can be social, emotional or a combination of all three, such as the birth of your children. Milestones can be further subcategorized into pleasant (losing your virginity; getting your driver's license), unpleasant (death of a parent) or totally unremarkable (first bank account), depending on your point of view. If our culture had a tradition of oral history richer than taunts such as "First comes love, then comes marriage, then comes a baby in the baby carriage," we might approach our milestones with less foreboding. For example, who among us honestly looks forward to going "over the hill"—turning 40, feeling our physical prowess decline and breathing our last breath? Wouldn't it be better if we could approach our fifth decade anticipating the perspective, wisdom and mastery of skills that come with the post-mid-life package?

In *The Seasons of a Man's Life,* Daniel J. Levinson writes that each era in a man's life "has its own distinctive and unifying qualities." The Talmud, Confucius and the Greek poet and lawmaker Solon have offered similar sentiments. At the risk of trivializing 2,500 years of scholarly work on mapping men's milestones, we'd like to offer our condensed version of life's road atlas. All milestones don't happen in the same order or at the same age for everyone—marriage and first child, for instance. But others can't be rearranged, such as marriage, divorce and second marriage. And some milestones get skipped altogether. What we're saying is the map isn't carved in stone, but if you can nod your head in agreement with a few of the markers you've already passed, perhaps you can find solace in reading about the ones you've yet to encounter. A map—even one as vague as this—beats a taunt any day.

BIRTH TO PUBERTY

Childhood developmental psychology is practically its own branch of science, so we'll just mention a few of the more significant events.

How about circumcision? Religious or secular, Mr.

Happy takes on a new look forever. More universally, there are memorable events such as cutting your first tooth, losing your first tooth, your first day of school, learning to count to 100, the first time riding your bike without training wheels and your first ejaculation, which marks the biological onset of puberty. Wasn't that a busy decade?

Our society is fond of making a fuss over puberty while ignoring what's really happening. Modern American male puberty rites include first communion, bar mitzvah, confirmation, getting a Social Security card and bank account, taking on a paper route and other such tedious chores. None of our puberty rites has much to do with ejaculating, which is probably just as well, since ejaculating is exciting enough in its own right. Still, I think I would have enjoyed a weekend at a brothel more than daydreaming about it in confirmation class. But puberty could have been worse. Bantu natives of North Kavirondo are circumcised without anesthesia at puberty and thrown into solitary confinement to heal and ponder the hardships of life. By comparison, confirmation class wasn't so bad.

TEENS

Trials outnumber errors only marginally in this decade. The good news is we can have sex. The bad news is we can't think of much else. The social consequence of this biological directive is an overwhelming tendency for us to make decisions with our smaller heads, leading us to actions that propel us toward and through most teenage milestones.

This is the age of your first kiss. Nearly as monumental is the "driving firsts" trilogy: first time behind the wheel, first license and first solo drive. Only then are you equipped to move on to the biological/emotional/social event of first sex in a car. Quite possibly, this can also be your last sex in a car, depending on how tall you are, how big your car is, how easily your legs cramp and how diligent the local police are at patrolling teenage parking spots.

Few horrors of this awkward epoch are as unnerving as high-school graduation. At age 17 or 18, you are expected to come up with a coherent, socially acceptable plan for your entire life and recite it dutifully to your relatives, your parents' friends and an endless string of college admissions officers. And heaven help you if you fail to follow any part of the program to the letter. (College admissions officers have this special facial gesture—more like a nervous tic, actually—reserved for "After college, I'd really like to drive to L.A. and play guitar in a rock band.")

Not surprisingly, many of us experience our first serious hangover around this time. Learning to handle alcohol is a trial-and-error thing, and few escape without at least one forever-memorable night spent gripping the sides of a toilet bowl with white-knuckled attention.

If there's anything positive to remember about passing from high school to the rest of your life, it's this: You'll never again look as goofy as you did for your senior-class photo.

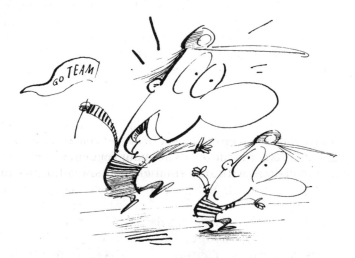

Take Your Dad to the Park

For Father's Day, don't just take your dad to your local Steak 'n' Suds; take him to a ballgame. A study from Ball State University finds that older folks who just *watch* sporting events feel better about themselves than those who don't. The study looked at 500 people over age 60 to see what influenced happiness. Involvement in sports—playing or just watching—ranked right up there, right after health and income.

TWENTIES

The Talmud's "Sayings of the Fathers" marks age 20 as the time for seeking a livelihood. Most of us graduate from college at least once in our 20s, and a fair number of us score entry level jobs that an older person wouldn't touch with a ten-foot pole. We think we're so cool in our 20s.

Solon said the years from 21 to 28 "ripen to completeness the powers of a man, and his worth becomes plain to see."

My former roommate, Russ—a philosopher in his own right—said, "Everything we do in life, we do in order to get laid," which, I believe, holds most true for men in their 20s. In this decade we combine our newfound aura of worth and the hormonal momentum of our teens to rent our first apartments, buy our first sporty new cars and set about trying to have sex as often as we can. This sexual conquest may even lead to love and marriage, but not necessarily in that order.

The harbingers of mid-life can begin to appear as age 30 approaches—your first gray hair, your first purchase of "full-cut" jeans for "the comfortable adult lifestyle" and your first major promotion to a position directing fresh college grads in jobs you wouldn't touch with a ten-foot pole.

THIRTIES

Confucius said, "At 30 I had planted my feet firm upon the ground." My dad said his 30s were some of the best years of his life. His career was blossoming, he still had the health and strength of a young man, he owned a decent home with my mom, and his kids were old enough to be interesting but not so old as to be uninterested in doing things with him. But I'm not my dad.

Since my old roomie, Russ, also told me "Nobody expects you to be responsible in your 20s," I crossed the threshold of full-on adulthood with much trepidation. According to the youthful rhetoric of the 1960s (I was only 10 when Woodstock happened, but my ears were fully developed), 30 is the age at which I would become untrustworthy. I, of course, like the rest of the baby boomer generation, resolved much of my anxiety about turning 30 by disowning this view. I now find the 30s just fine.

I'll be 33 by the time you read this. After a false start in my early 20s, I'm four years into a successful marriage, six years into a successful career, my wife and I just bought our second house, and we plan to have kids soon. Although I've sprouted a few gray hairs and my body has become too efficient to burn all the calories I'd like to feed it, I've never felt younger or more together. And I'm flattered when younger colleagues or students on the high-school cross-country ski team that I coach seek my counsel. The only really frightening milestone you have to face in your 30s is turning 35—the point at which you realize the legal age for becoming president is much too low.

FORTIES

You rarely hear the word "mid-life" without "crisis" immediately after. Why? The bad news about mid-life is you can't ejaculate as many times in a day as you could during your teens and 20s. The good news is you don't have to. We interpret this phenomenon, coupled with graying hair, rising forehead and loss of waistline, as the onset of biological decline. We're starting to die. Perhaps. But depending on how you look at it, we're also just starting to live. The next two decades have the potential to be your greatest—or so I've heard.

Age 40 is "for understanding," according to the Talmud. Confucius said, "At 40 I no longer suffered from perplexities." From 42 to 56, Solon said, "the tongue and the mind for 14 years together are now at their best." And Russ said, "You won't really get your s—t together until you're 40," which is pretty much what everyone else said, though much less straightforwardly.

Mid-life is the time when we ask ourselves "Is that all there is?" then either say "Yes, thank you" or set out to do more. Few of us can pass the mid-life transition without some sort of upheaval.

If you spent your 20s and 30s chasing after someone else's dreams—partnership in the firm, house in the 'burbs, wife, 2.3 children and a station wagon with fake wood on the sides—you may be in for a rough time. "At 40, you look at the life you've created and decide 'Do I like it?' " says Ron Levant, Ed.D., psychologist and coauthor of *Between Father and Child*. If the answer is no, career changes, divorce, moving and remarriage can all be milestone by-products of mid-life transition. But even if you're satisfied with what you have, you may still find yourself dipping into the kids' college fund for a motorcycle, an electric guitar or a trip to the Himalayas while chanting the mid-life mantra "If I don't do it now, I'll never do it."

Once you're through the rough surf at the shore of mid-life and dedicated, or rededicated, to what you're doing, there'll be no stopping you. But turning 40 is no guarantee of

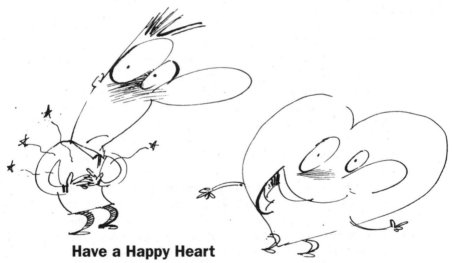

Have a Happy Heart

Treating depression may play a key role in preventing and treating cardiovascular disease, says George Kaplan, Ph.D., of the California Department of Health Services in Berkeley. He found that depression seems to compound the effects of smoking and high blood cholesterol. Depressed men who smoked, for example, had nearly triple the thickening of the walls of the carotid arteries (the ones that nourish the brain) as men who smoked but were not depressed. So beating the chronic blues may be yet another step on the road toward avoiding stroke and heart attack.

success. Some men are locked in mid-life crisis forever. In your 40s you can either accept yourself as you are or continue to wonder why a major-league baseball team didn't offer you a contract. If you choose the second route, gold chains, liposuction, Porsches and trophy wives constitute the milestones from here on in.

FIFTIES

In most models of the male life cycle, the 50s are simply a continuation of the 40s. Plato makes one distinction in Book 10 of *The Republic,* in which he claims no one is old enough to have wisdom until he's 50. But he also notes that turning 50 offers no assurance of that. They must have had gold chains, trophy wives and Porsches back then, too.

The silly antics of Donald Trump types are well documented in the tabloids, but they're far from the norm. "Most men just don't do this," says Nolan Brohaugh, M.S.W., senior associate at the Menninger Clinic in Topeka, Kansas. "They find other ways of making the transition—often by recognizing that it's time to give something back to society. Many become interested in mentoring or teaching."

This passing of the torch is a milestone that has its own satisfactions. "One generation of men, through its own example, has always prepared the next generation to recognize its possibilities in life," says Brohaugh.

SIXTIES

Of a man aged 56 to 63, Solon said, "Still . . . is he able, but never so nimble in speech and wit as he was in the days of his prime." For many men, retirement is the major milestone of the 60s. "Having paid his dues to society, he has earned the right to be and do what is most important to himself," says Levinson.

The kids have grown, and you don't have a job to keep you planted in one place, so you're free to travel or move someplace pleasant. But don't go so far away that you can't visit your grandchildren—those little conduits of revenge that you can spoil in retaliation for all the crap your kids put you through.

Instead of sitting in a rocker and waiting to die, many retired men turn to new careers—often in artistic or humanitarian fields that younger people can't afford to pursue without great economic sacrifice. Jimmy Carter builds houses for the homeless. My dad joined the Coast Guard Auxiliary and drives disabled people to their doctors' appointments for the Red Cross. Mikhail Gorbachev has a successful consulting business. You're only as useless as you want to be in your 60s. And if you want to be really useless, you can always take up golf.

SEVENTIES

The Bible suggests that three score and ten is long enough for any man to walk the face of the earth. Most other life-cycle scholars quit here, too. But some modern exceptions were deep into a second career at age 70, or even 80. Novelist James Michener is now lecturing at the University of South Florida; schoolteacher Grandma Moses expanded the limits of primitive-style oil painting during her retirement; and everybody knows what B-movie actor Ronald Reagan did. (We just don't know why.)

"You're only as old as you feel" is a cliché, but only because it smacks of truth. Sure, men in their 70s have a greater share of physical maladies than younger men— prostate problems, arthritis, forgetfulness and, uh, something else, to name but a few. But many of these degenerative maladies can be avoided in our 70s if we take care of ourselves now. Since we started with a cliché, let's end with one: "If you don't change the path you're on right now, you'll eventually get to where you're headed." Set the groundwork now for a healthful eighth decade, and you might make it. Don't, and you probably won't.

If you're willing and able to go on from here, you do so without a map. But be a pal and take some trip notes for the rest of us who'd like to get there, too.

—Don Cuerdon

Part 5

WOMEN AND SEX

Long-Distance Lust

A long and happy life is a long and sexy life.
Here's rock-solid advice on how to
boost your sex drive at any age.

● ● ● ● ● ● ● ● ● ● ● ● ● ● ● ● ● ● ●

WHEN YOU'RE 20 and you have trouble getting an erection, you can shrug it off as nerves or too much beer at the frat party. When you're 40 and the same thing happens, you wonder if it's the end of a long and rewarding sexual career. You've heard the conventional wisdom: After 40, or even during one's 30s, sex drive heads south; erections start balking, and when they rise, they're flying at only half-mast. In other words, like many a man's hair, male sexuality recedes and eventually disappears.

The conventional wisdom is wrong. Aging does bring some sexual changes, but they're minor. The fact is, sexual vitality is largely independent of age. If you want a great love life at 45 or 55, or 85 for that matter, you can have it.

Here's another common myth we're going to blow out of the water: Men don't peak sexually at 18. What the research actually shows, according to *The Kinsey Institute New Report on Sex,* is only that men's sexual *daydreaming* peaks then.

When asked how often they had sexual thoughts, young men aged 12 to 19 said they thought about sex every five minutes; men in their 40s said they had sexual thoughts about every half-hour. So guys in their 40s who think about sex 30 times a day aren't exactly shriveling up. And one reason teens daydream about sex so much (besides having so much time to kill in math class) is that they're less likely to *have* sex routinely available to them.

And when we talk about staying sexually active, we're not just talking about baby boomers here. A University of Chicago survey of 6,000 married couples over age 60 showed that 37 percent had sex at least once a week.

But don't men lose their erections as they grow older? There's another myth in serious need of debunking. Experts estimate that only about 5 percent of 40-year-olds suffer erection problems; at 65, the figure is 15 to 25 percent. Most of it is caused not by sexual difficulties but rather by medical conditions such as diabetes and by drug treatment of other non-sexual conditions. "Erection problems," says John C. Beck, M.D., a gerontologist at the University of California, Los Angeles, "are not a natural part of aging."

SEX IS LIFELONG

Evolution endowed us with a lifelong capacity to reproduce. But of course, we're not 18 forever. What really happens sexually as we age? For otherwise healthy men, surprisingly little. Aging brings a slow decline in production of testosterone, the hormone responsible for men's sex drive. But most men produce much more of this hormone than they need anyway. Even late in life, when testosterone levels are on the low side, they're still usually within the normal range. And the hardware itself remains virtually unchanged. "If I showed you a photograph of a man's erection at 20 and at 80, you would not be able to tell the difference," says urologist Dudley Seth Danoff, M.D., author of the book *Superpotency.*

So now you know the good news. Does that mean you're guaranteed to stay potent until they carry you away? Not necessarily. But there are a number of things you can do to ensure that your sex life stays vital and vigorous.

Relax, then get excited. Too much stress is hell on the libido. In an admittedly bizarre study at the University of Utah, psychologists wired the penises of 54 volunteers, aged 21 to 46, with an instrument that measures erection, then showed them X-rated videos and recorded their arousal levels. Some of the volunteers were then wired with a new fake electrode and were told that at some point during a repeat showing of the sex videos, they would receive a painful, but harmless, electrical shock. Guess what happened. Right: Arousal plunged 35 percent in those expecting a shock.

Stress works its sexual mischief in two ways. It triggers the fight-or-flight reflex, which sends blood away from the central body (and penis) out to the limbs to supply the muscles involved in self-defense and escape. It also stimulates the secretion of cortisol, a natural chemical that suppresses production of sex hormones. "The message is 'Relax,'" says Louanne Cole, Ph.D., a San Francisco sex therapist. "You'll feel more aroused, and your erections will stand up better." To relax your way into great lovemaking, try a hot bath or shower beforehand—either solo or with your partner. In addition to setting the stage for good sex, hot baths increase blood flow into the penis.

Simmer all day and cook all night. Try a technique called "simmering," suggests sex therapist Bernie Zilbergeld, Ph.D. Most men have moments of sexual arousal several times a day: the beauty in the Corvette on the way to work, the cute waitress at lunch, the sexy ad in a magazine and the phone call from the client with that Kathleen Turner voice. You can hold on to those zingy moments by simmering, which Dr. Zilbergeld describes in his book *The New Male Sexuality*. Whenever you have a sexual feeling toward a woman, go ahead and focus on it for a few moments. Let yourself fantasize about her, guilt-free. Then let go of the thought. An hour later, return to it and relive it. Continue replaying your fantasies every few hours, but as you get ready to go home, substitute your steady for your fantasy ladies. Simmering keeps feelings of arousal bubbling away until you and your lover are ready to make them boil.

Try a natural aphrodisiac. For centuries, oysters have had a reputation for being aphrodisiacs. While oysters contain no magic sex-enhancing ingredient, they *are* high in the mineral zinc, an important component of semen and the prostate gland. Men with moderate to severe zinc deficiencies may suffer impaired libido and low sperm counts, according to Sheldon Saul Hendler, M.D., Ph.D., assistant clinical professor of medicine at the University of California, San Diego. Other foods rich in zinc include lean meats, seafood, whole-grain products and wheat germ. No other specific foods hold a promise of sexual ecstasy, but one diet does. It's the same low-fat, low-cholesterol diet the American Heart Association (AHA) recommends to prevent heart attack. In addition to keeping off extra pounds, the AHA diet may prevent the clogging of the arteries that supply blood to both the heart and the penis. A low-fat diet might help sex drive in another way as well. A recent study by endocrinologist A. Wayne Meikle, M.D., of the University of Utah showed that four hours after consuming a high-fat meal, participants' testosterone levels dropped 30 percent, possibly enough in some cases to dampen sex drive.

Stay sensitive. One significant age-related change in the penis is a gradual loss of sensitivity to touch, because as the years pass, the nerves in the penis lose some ability to transmit stimulation to the brain. One way to compensate, says sexual medicine specialist Theresa Crenshaw, M.D., of the Crenshaw Clinic in San Diego, is to use a sexual lubricant. In recent years, science has produced several new ones that feel slicker and less messy than the long-time commercial leader K-Y jelly. Check in your drugstore for Probe, Astroglide and other inventively named sexual lubricants.

Get aerobic, get erotic. Want to work up more sexual energy at any age? Then work up a good sweat. Recently, University of California researchers studied 95 out-of-shape men, average age 47. Seventeen took little strolls for one hour three days a week, while 78 got sweaty in more strenuous aerobic workouts.

After nine months, the strollers reported no change in sexual desire or activity and an increase in sex problems. But the aerobic group reported a jump in sexual desire, a 30 percent increase in frequency of intercourse, fewer sex problems and more pleasure from orgasm.

Harvard anthropologist Philip Whitten, Ph.D., came to the same conclusion in a study of male swimmers aged 40 to 69. Those in their 40s reported sex about seven times a month—almost twice a week. That's about 40 percent more sex than the average man in his 40s has, according to *The Janus Report on Sexual Behavior.*

Be strong where it counts. Any moderate regular exercise adds to sexual longevity, but one particular exercise actually boosts the intensity of orgasm. Known as Kegels, after Arnold Kegel, M.D., the doctor who popularized it, this intimate workout strengthens the pubococcygeus (or PC) muscle that runs from the base of the penis to the tailbone. To do a Kegel, squeeze the same muscles you would use to stop the flow of urine. Do a set of ten contractions several times a day. Within a few weeks, you should notice that your orgasms feel more intense and pleasurable.

Lose a little weight. Ronette L. Kolotkin, Ph.D., of the Duke University Diet and Fitness Center, surveyed the effects of weight loss on 64 participants, average age mid-40s. The study is still in progress, but her preliminary results are revealing: "Moderate weight loss (10 to 30 pounds) significantly improved the sexual desire and feelings of attractiveness," Dr. Kolotkin says.

Coffee keeps things hot. When researchers at the University of Michigan surveyed 744 married couples aged 60 or older, they discovered that the daily coffee drinkers among them were almost twice as likely to describe themselves as "sexually active"—62 percent versus 38 percent of the noncoffee drinkers. Coffee-drinking men also reported fewer erection problems. The reason for the connection isn't yet understood.

Don't mix sex with these drugs. Moderate amounts of stimulants may arouse the libido, but many other drugs do the opposite, says James Goldberg, Ph.D., research director at the Damlugi Bari Clinic in San Diego. The main offenders are:

■ Blood pressure medications, especially the so-called calcium channel blockers, such as Procardia and Calan.

■ Most tranquilizers, especially Librium but also Valium and Xanax.

■ Any pain relievers containing codeine.

■ Most antidepressant drugs, with the exception of some of the newer types, such as Wellbutrin.

■ Anti-epileptic drugs such as Dilantin.

■ Ulcer and other stomach disorder drugs such as Tagamet and Reglan.

If you experience sexual problems and are using any of these medications, consult your doctor. A lower dosage or a switch to an alternative medication may get you back in the game.

● ●

Potency Zappers

Following an 18-month study, a Cairo University professor has discovered a link between wearing polyester underwear and impotence. The professor blames the static electricity generated by the polyester material. Consider yourself warned.

Nonprescription medications can also make your libido go slack: "If the label says 'May cause drowsiness,' it's probably a sex offender," Dr. Crenshaw says. These include many cold and flu formulas, some allergy products and motion sickness drugs.

Go easy on the booze if you want to boogie. Alcohol is probably the world's most sex-dampening drug. It may relax inhibitions, but beyond that first drink, alcohol becomes a central nervous system depressant that impairs libido, erection and sexual pleasure. A general rule is that the amount of alcohol it takes to affect your driving ability (for an average-size man, anything more than two drinks in an hour) can also affect your libido, says Dr. Goldberg.

Stand by your woman. So you're envious of your bachelor friends? Don't be. Your sex life will be a lot better if you work on tending your own garden than if you try your hand playing the field. According to *The Janus Report on Sexual Behavior,* couples are more sexually active than singles. Forty-seven percent of singles described themselves as sexually active to very sexually active. Among couples, the figure was 54 percent. And almost 60 percent of those in couples said that sex had improved after marriage.

If marriage enhances sex, divorce often crushes it. Researchers at Wayne State University extracted data on the sex lives of 340 divorced people from a large national sample and found that over a year's time, one-quarter were celibate, and only one-quarter made love more than once a week. "Divorce is depressing," says Dr. Cole, "and depression impairs libido."

In the end, though, demography works to older men's sexual advantage. On average, women live longer than men. Not generally the best of news for us, but if we stay fit and eat right, we can reap the rewards at the end. At age 65, there are 1.25 women for every man. By age 80, women outnumber men 2 to 1. Stay healthy and sexually active long enough, and you'll live to see what the Beach Boys discovered in Surf City—two girls for every boy.

—Michael Castleman

Female Sex Secrets

*If women could give us love lessons, here are the
secrets they would want to teach us first.*

●●●●●●●●●●●●●●●●●●●

THIS IS WHERE you put 'it' in," she said.

Twelve years ago, Todd, Geoff and I were three
Midwesterners just out of college, living in a fourth-floor
walk-up on the fringes of Greenwich Village. We had moved
to New York City to begin careers, and we were taking our
first awkward steps in this new world. I suppose the same
could be said about our first relationships with women.

One night around midnight, we got to talking about
women, sex and women's bodies. In a way it was typical
guy talk for men in their early 20s, except that there was a
woman present, a girlfriend of Todd's. One of us had con-
fessed to having trouble figuring women out "down there,"
so in service to us (and perhaps to other women), she
opened a spiral-bound notebook and drew a circle, followed by three smaller circles arranged vertically inside
the first one.

It was then, indicating the largest of the three inner circles, that she told us where to put it. We were transfixed.
"And this is where we go to the bathroom," she continued,
pointing to the circle just above it. "Because they're so close,
sex, and even petting, hurts us sometimes. It's also why we
get so many damn infections." We hadn't even gotten to the
clitoris when it occurred to me: If we, three college-educated
adult men living in the big city, needed help with the basics
of women's bodies, what about other men?

It's not that we didn't have any girlfriends of our own.
After all, this was before AIDS was an issue, and we were
young and single in a city teeming with available women.
But as the impromptu anatomy lesson demonstrated, we had
a lot to learn.

Now in my mid-30s, I'm a veteran of several long-term
relationships as well as some more brief entanglements, but
I've yet to marry.

WHAT DO WOMEN WANT IN BED?

And I still find myself asking questions. Indeed, I often think that the power to read minds, were it available, would be best appreciated in the bedroom. Just imagine if each time you made love to a woman she knew exactly what you wanted as soon as, or even before, you did. And imagine that you knew exactly what she wanted. There'd be no need to ask, to take that risk of saying or doing the wrong thing.

Fortunately, as a journalist I can ask questions on the job, even the intimate questions that men often keep to themselves. But in my quest to learn more about the minds and bodies of women, I had another factor working in my favor—they wanted to talk. Like Todd's girlfriend from our Greenwich Village days, the women I interviewed about sex were delighted by the opportunity to reveal the secrets they've always wished men knew, even if they were afraid to tell them to their own lovers.

While no book or magazine article can claim to be exhaustive on so complex a topic, following are the six sexual secrets women volunteered most frequently.

1. She's starved for praise. A woman's body image can bring her more torment (or pleasure) than most men ever realize. Part of the reason is sociological: Women who subscribe to social and media norms feel compelled to look "appealing, earthy, sensual, sexual, virginal, innocent, reliable, daring, mysterious, coquettish and thin," in the words of author Susie Orbach. Countless women pursue a kind of physical perfection that is impossible to achieve. It's not surprising, perhaps, that up to 200,000 women underwent breast augmentation surgery in 1989 alone and that at least 10 million women are affected by eating disorders.

In light of this vast aesthetic uncertainty among today's women, men need to recognize that praising a lover's beauty doesn't just boost her ego, it makes her feel comfortable.

Speaking of the best lovers in her life, Judy H., a graduate student, says, "It's not just what they did but how relaxed they made me feel. They made me confident about my body. And they made me feel really loved."

"The sounds of silence make it real hard to relax," adds Pat H., 27, a single artist from New England. "Talking is important, even if it's just someone saying 'I really find you attractive' or 'You're so soft.' Or if he says my name. I want to see his tender side."

"When I'm having sex with someone, I'm aware of where his eyes go and whether or not he wants the lights off," says Sharon L., 31, once divorced, from Providence, Rhode Island. "If a man gets up and turns the lights off, I take that to mean he doesn't want to see my body. As sexually confident as I am, it's not the same with my body. If a man isn't responsive, I withdraw. It's that simple.

"I think it's harder being a woman," she adds, "because we're worrying about breast size, fat thighs, stomach rolls and wrinkles. You want them to make you feel that none of it matters. I think in our hearts, everyone wants to be told she's beautiful."

2. Be twice as gentle as you think you should be. Sometimes, even as we strive to please, we men can come on too strong. One of the most important leaps a man can make sexually is to realize that what he feels below his waist is not what his partner feels. In fact, women may feel very little through the walls of the vagina most of the time because the nerve cells located along the vaginal walls are not all that plentiful. (And the clitoris, as we all know, the nerve center of female pleasure, is located outside the vagina.)

So what may be most pleasurable for a man—the deep, thrusting, in-and-out motions of intercourse—may provide very little sexual satisfaction for a woman. She may prefer woman-on-top positions, in which she can more carefully direct the thrusts toward stimulating her clitoris. Or she may prefer shallow penetration and positions in which the tip of the penis rides along the outer edges of the vagina, where the most excitation, nerve response and swelling naturally occur.

"I think the biggest mistake men make is that they touch you as hard as they want you to touch them," says Judy H. "It just doesn't work that way."

3. Learn to linger. This may be fundamental. Think of Mae West, arch–sex symbol of the 1930s who sang the praises of "A Guy What Takes His Time": "I don't like a big commotion/I'm a demon for slow motion" were just a few of the lyrics that shocked many people by revealing the long-suppressed truth about female sexuality. Even in our relatively enlightened time, speed remains an issue. While the occasional "quickie" can be as thrilling for our mates as it is for us, women usually find that rushed sex is bad sex.

The reason? Beyond emotional needs, women simply take longer than men to climax.

The experience of Ann M., 22, of Madison, Wisconsin, is typical in this sense. She had been sexually active for six years before she actually began to enjoy intercourse in a relationship that made her feel physically comfortable and "adult," orgasm and all.

Speaking of the man who opened her eyes to the erotic possibilities, she says, "It really helped that he was so patient."

Judy H. made a similar discovery. "I never had an orgasm till I was 20, even though I'd already slept with a lot of people," she says. The change came with a boyfriend, John, who patiently spent enough time with her to make her relax completely. For the first time she didn't feel as though she had to rush, even though she took a lot longer to climax than her partner.

In short, Ann and Judy found lovers who, in the words of Mae West, "would condescend to linger a while." And for them, that made all the difference.

4. Discover her secret pleasures. Compared with the male body, which betrays its arousal even when clothed, the female body retains an air of subtlety, even mystery. Witness the confusion surrounding the clitoris—among women as well as men.

A number of women I spoke to admitted not knowing even where to find their clitorises until more experienced, or possibly better read, boyfriends showed them.

"When I started dating in the early 1950s, almost none of my sexual partners seemed to know what or where a clitoris was," says Alice W., 48, a married writer from the Midwest. "Sometimes I thought I didn't have one or it was in the wrong place."

When a woman is aroused, a number of things normally happen. She experiences clitoral swelling, a flush about the chest and neck, sweating and nipple erection. When doctors or sexologists speak of "clitoral erection," they're referring to the head of the clitoris and the immediate surrounding area, which is composed of erectile tissue. Surrounding this sensitive tissue are nerve endings that, in the right hands (and with the right stimulation), can greatly increase a woman's pleasure.

It's also worth knowing that as orgasm approaches, the clitoris momentarily shrinks out of sight, burrowing back beneath its hood. This may confuse many men, who see it as a sign of sexual turnoff when in fact, at this stage, it's a sign of intense arousal.

5. If you question, so will she. It's here that my wish for mind-reading powers returns with renewed urgency. For while it's obvious enough that women appreciate a lover who attends to their needs, questions such as "Does this feel good?" are not always welcome.

Teresa R., a single 25-year-old from the Midwest, says

• •

My Face or Yours?

Men and women not only think differently, we speak and gesture differently, according to the book *He Says, She Says* by Lillian Glass, Ph.D. She finds that even the smallest facial expressions are loaded with meaning.

Men

■ Tend to avoid eye contact and do not look directly at the other person

■ Tilt their heads to the side and look at the other person from an angle when listening to a conversation

■ Frown and squint when listening

■ Provide fewer facial expressions in feedback and fewer reactions

Women

■ Look more directly at another person and have better eye contact

■ Look at the other person directly facing them, with their heads and eyes facing forward when listening

■ Smile and nod when listening

■ Provide more facial expressions in feedback and more reactions that sometimes plain talk works in bed, sometimes not. "Women today are not as afraid to say what does and does not feel good," she says. "But when I tell my boyfriend something doesn't feel good—when he puts his finger in a certain place in my vagina, for example—it makes me feel like I'm at the gynecologist."

Karla D., a 28-year-old secretary from Philadelphia, says she wishes men were more adventurous with her body. But there are times when she feels like having sex without needing to "teach" a partner in bed. When one man said "Karla, tell me what makes you feel wonderful," she was glad he asked but at the same time wished he didn't have to. When told that that kind of question is tough for the average man to ask, she says, "Trying to come up with an answer is hard, too. I mean, I'm not trying to make it scientific."

In her latest book, *Women on Top,* Nancy Friday says: "Men might learn if women told them exactly what they wanted. But women hate giving instructions to the man, telling him what to do, what it is they want; getting involved in their own seduction makes them too responsible, breaks the mood of being swept away."

So where does that leave us poor men who aim to please but don't always know how? Perhaps Elyse A., 26, of New York City has the right idea. "It would help if men knew a woman has more nerve endings on the outside of her body than on the inside," she says. "They can learn it by sensing what the other person is doing while they're touching. You don't always have to explain it."

Judy H. recalls that her boyfriend John changed her usually detached reaction to receiving oral sex by exploring her genitals carefully, by watching—feeling—her body's reactions to his motions and by spending enough time with her that she felt she could relax completely.

In sex, then, the best communication may be nonverbal. A man needs to read a woman's body rather than always rely on her to put her wishes into words.

6. Once you know the rules, break them. While learning all the ins and outs of intercourse can do a lot for one's sex life, there is a subtle danger of becoming obsessed with performance and technique, of trying too hard.

"Some men think 'I'll do this for ten minutes, then that for ten minutes, then roll her over,' " says Eleanor H., 34, a legal assistant from South Carolina. "Are they reading this in a magazine? They want their partner to go back to her friends and say 'John really knew what to do.' "

"I've had two guys who were amazing," says Terri D., 26, once engaged but never married. "They taught me that having sex isn't an exercise, that there's so much potential. And yet some men look at it as piecework, step-by-step, then orgasm, then you go to sleep."

"I guess at 22 I had a list of 'performing' things," says Sandi L., 28, a physical therapist from Cleveland. "Now I don't give a hoot about them. There's no list. Whatever happens that day happens. And it's more enjoyable in that there's no A, then B, then C. It never gets boring."

Needless to say, when men are excessively concerned with performance, they tend to spoil the fun for themselves as well as for their partners. "Accused of being selfish, men are not really selfish enough," says Paul Pearsall, Ph.D., in his bestseller *Super Marital Sex.* "For they are too busy trying to do instead of be and experience. Love becomes a product they try to 'make.' "

While being spontaneous carries a certain amount of risk, it can also lead to the greatest satisfaction. Knowledge is better than ignorance. But sometimes the thrill of discovery is best left to the participants.

—Curtis Pesman

Shape Up Your Sex Life

How to keep that sex machine of yours
mechanically sound for a long, long time.

•••••••••••••••••••

JOSEPH KHOURY RUNS A COUPLE OF MILES every morning, eats a low-fat diet and swims for a half-hour most days to relieve stress. While it's a routine that will certainly keep his heart strong and his mind clear, he has another motive, something most guys in their mid-30s don't think about but should.

"I've never had a problem with erectile function, and I don't plan on having one either, because I'm doing something about it now," says Khoury. Now it's only fair to point out here that Khoury is not your average health-minded guy. He's a urologist at Georgetown University Medical Center in Washington, D.C. Which is to say he's studied the equipment responsible for producing erections and he's observed what happens when men take care of the equipment...and what happens when they don't.

Few of us are as forward-thinking as Dr. Khoury. We take a lot of things for granted, especially when we're young and seemingly omnipotent. Right through our 20s, we didn't have to work out as often to stay muscular. We ate whatever we wanted and didn't gain weight. And we never thought twice about getting an erection. If anything was a problem in that department, it was getting one too often. "All you needed was a girl to walk by in a tight sweater," says John Mulcahy, M.D., a professor of urology at the Indiana University Medical Center in Indianapolis. "And at night, the penis would get as hard as a piece of plastic pipe."

But now that many of us have passed the age of 30, business might not be as usual. We already know that as our metabolism slows down, it takes more time in the gym to maintain our muscle tone. Most of us can't indulge in certain foods the way we used to without bulging at the waistline.

And guess what? "Whenever things start to go to pot in your body, the erection will be no exception," says Dr. Mulcahy.

The basic science behind erectile function has emerged only in the last decade or so. And while the research is revealing that a complex interaction of hormones and brain chemicals is necessary, "all it really is is blood flow," says Dr. Mulcahy.

WHAT THE PENIS NEEDS

Just as the heart needs open blood vessels to receive an adequate supply of oxygen, the penis requires an open pathway to receive blood for an erection. And just as fat in the bloodstream can build blockages in the arteries of the heart, so can it build blockages in the arteries of the penis.

Studies of artery plaques show that they are present in our bodies as early as our teens. But as a rule they don't affect the function of the heart until after age 50, when heart attack rates escalate in men. However, because some blood vessels to the penis are narrower, they may show signs of unhealthy living earlier.

According to the experts, the average man in his 30s will begin to notice that his erections aren't quite as firm as they used to be and that they don't respond to those tight sweaters as rapidly. And thanks to the added stress we carry as we climb the career ladder and begin raising families, the odds are greater that moments will occur when our penises say no while our brains say yes.

It doesn't have to be that way. In fact, if you look at studies of men who stay fit and trim and who know how to relieve stress, you see little if any decline in erectile function through middle age. "Theoretically, there is no reason for your potency to change as you age," says Dr. Khoury, who knows men in their 80s who still have sex three times a week. The one thing they have in common: They took care of themselves better than most men. "I believe this could be a big incentive for keeping fit," says Dr. Mulcahy.

Where to start? According to the experts, if you smoke, quitting tops the list of advice for improving sexual fitness. Cigarette smoking accelerates the formation of blockages in the heart's arteries, and there's every reason to believe that it does the same to the vessels that supply blood to the penis. In fact, smoking is now considered a major factor in erectile dysfunction, with the first signs of harm appearing by age 40.

Besides leading to plaque buildup along artery walls, nicotine in tobacco is also a blood vessel constrictor. That means each puff makes it more difficult for blood to get to the penis when it's stimulated. When men stop smoking, Dr. Mulcahy says, most will get firmer erections. It's a subtle improvement, and some smokers don't realize they have a problem until they quit.

AEROBIC SEX

Second on the list is to develop an aerobic exercise routine. The more fit you become as a result of exercise, the more sex you'll have, and the better it will be, says a study published in the *Archives of Sexual Behavior*. They're not just talking *perceived* better. They're talking more orgasms. In the study, 78 healthy but inactive men began aerobic exercise three to five days a week for an hour each time. A control group simply walked at a moderate pace three to five days a week. During the study, each man kept a diary of sexual activity. The results showed that the sex lives of the aerobic exercisers significantly improved. The more they exercised, the more and better sex they had. Meanwhile, the sex lives of the walkers changed very little.

It doesn't matter which type of aerobic exercise you choose, as long as you do it a minimum of two to three times each week and stick with it for at least 20 minutes per session. Running and rowing are both good choices.

When it comes to diet, the bottom line is limiting your fat intake. Again, the logic goes that what's good for the arteries supplying blood flow to the heart will also be good for those supplying blood to the penis.

How much fat you can safely consume is still under debate. While the American Heart Association recommends less than 30 percent of daily calorie intake from fat for the average man, Dr. Khoury argues that a "high-potency" diet ought to be approximately 20 percent calories from fat.

Limiting fat in your diet also reduces weight gain, and

according to Dr. Mulcahy, excess pounds can actually make critical inches of the penis disappear. Informal studies he has done of obese men show that—up to a point—a man will regain one inch of his penis for every 35 pounds of weight lost. Not a bad incentive for someone who's really heavy. But more practically, keeping your weight down will reduce the risk of high blood pressure and diabetes, both of which impair the ability to have an erection. Keeping blood pressure normal also means avoiding antihypertension drugs, which can cause impotence.

STRESS LEAVES YOU LIMP

While not smoking, staying fit and eating right will avert problems down the road, mental stress is probably the greatest cause of erection trouble now, says Jack Jaffe, M.D., director of the Potency Recovery Center in Van Nuys, California. "In our society we're under stress throughout the entire day, and our sex lives tend to suffer later in the evening," he says.

It was not easy to find men willing to recount a story about such an experience. But after much wheedling, a friend

. . . .

Delaying Tactic

Good news for the 20 to 30 million American men who suffer from premature ejaculation: The antidepressant drug Prozac has a side effect of delaying orgasm, and it may one day be prescribed for premature ejaculation. In an experiment, 46 men who were unable to have active sex for even 30 seconds before orgasm were given 20 to 80 milligrams of Prozac daily. At the end of the study, all of them were able to have intercourse for longer than five minutes. Furthermore, when these men stopped taking the drug, they did not revert to premature ejaculation. It's not that Prozac lowers sex drive, explains research leader Roger Crenshaw, M.D., of La Jolla, California. Rather, it raises the threshold at which men ejaculate by increasing the amount of a naturally occurring brain chemical associated with the process. He noted that Prozac does not affect the mental state of someone with no depression. The treatment costs about $400 for doctor's fees plus roughly $60 a month for the drug, which is available only by prescription.

I'll call Frank, who lives in a town I'll call Baltimore, allowed as how he once had a problem in bed. It was at a time in his life when the stress was thick indeed. He'd been wrapped up in a bitter separation from his wife for months, bickering over money and custody of their child. After the divorce was final, he was amazed to meet a woman interested in a no-strings-attached arrangement. Following several weeks of getting to know each other, the time came for a particularly romantic evening. But during the hours before his date, Frank says he engaged in a rancid argument with his ex-wife over an upcoming weekend visit with his three-year-old son. The conversation stayed in his mind the entire evening.

"My girlfriend was dressed to kill, and she was in the mood," he says. "But all I could think about was how to strangle my ex-wife. Nothing was happening below the belt."

Dr. Mulcahy says it's common for stress to interfere with the ability to raise an erection. But he also says it's important to let the incident drop. Guys get into trouble when they worry that something terrible is wrong with the equipment and that the problem will recur. Then they get a recycling and magnification of the problem, which leads to performance anxiety. And the human brain being the practical joker that it is, if you expect trouble, you'll often find it.

The one thing you don't want to do is drink alcohol to relieve stress. Shakespeare probably said it best in *Macbeth* when he described alcohol as that which "provokes the desire, but . . . takes away the performance." For a more contemporary model, we have Jim Morrison, whose well-documented whiskey binges led him to write a poem entitled "Lament for the Death of My C—k."

Alcohol is a depressant that slows down reflexes, including sexual ones. Besides impairing immediate performance, alcohol, when consumed excessively for too long, can have a direct effect on the testicles, decreasing production of testosterone, upsetting the delicate balance of hormones and brain chemicals required to make an erection.

ACT YOUR AGE

Finally, however strong your potency is, there's no point in trying to compete with the 20-year-old you. You and your partner are bound to have a bit less spontaneity in your sex life than you had back then, if only because you have more on your mind, greater responsibilities, richer interests and a fuller schedule. Dr. Jaffe says the way to avoid psychological problems here that could interfere with your performance is not to wait for the magic moment. "You've got to make it happen," he says. "That may mean setting a date, sitting down to discuss what your needs are, whatever it takes."

Bottom line: A man's got to put some work into maintaining his youthful potency. But this ought not be a burden. Dr. Khoury sees it all as a kind of symphony. Staying fit makes you feel good and look good. Eating right and properly relieving stress give you energy: "It all coincides really quite elegantly. You run, you eat a good diet, you get a good body image, and you keep your mind at ease—all that ties into your sexuality," says Dr. Khoury. "It really is something worth working for."

—Tim Friend

Spread Pleasure

Take off your clothes together and rediscover the joys of the soft, caring touch. Learn the forgotten art of sensual massage.

• • • • • • • • • • • • • • • • • • •

"WITH A WARM, QUIET PLACE and a bottle of scented oil, you can spread pleasure over every inch of your partner's body," says Gordon Inkeles, best-selling author of *The Art of Sensual Massage.*

What a pity that we so seldom do it.

Even people who love each other and have been happily married for years tend to forget 95 percent of the vast and varied vocabulary of touch. After a few years of a relationship, the way we touch each other tends to be reduced to one of two things: We do it either in a completely sexless, perfunctory way (a peck on the cheek, a pat on the back) or in a way that is as sexual as you can get. Often when a man touches his mate at all, it's basically a way of asking a question: "Do you want to have sex?" First comes the touch, then the kiss, then a fast-forward to orgasm.

Even when we get sexual, the places that we touch each other tend to be limited to a couple of square inches of skin the dimensions of an airmail envelope. Whole kingdoms of the body, and of sensuous pleasure, go unnoticed. Says Inkeles: "It's entirely possible that a woman who's been married for years has never been touched behind the knee, or between the toes, by another adult since childhood." Our whole culture, in fact, is so starved for touch that sometimes people will have sex when all they really want is the feel and warmth of skin against skin.

NEVER TOO LATE

But it's never too late to learn the exquisite pleasures of touch and to rediscover each other in the process.

It's called *massage.*

Don't be intimidated by the word. There are types of massage that require lots of training and maybe even a few courses in human physiology, but that's not what we're talking about here. We're talking about simply using touch to give your partner pleasure and then to unashamedly *receive* it (which is also the goal of satisfying sex). That kind of touch doesn't take any particular training at all, although it does require that you care for each other.

Massage is a potent sex enhancer, says Inkeles, because it induces deep relaxation and rapidly dissipates the negative effects of stress. People tend to have sex as a way of relieving physical tension. But a far better approach is to slip into a state of deep relaxation *first,* through sensuous massage, and then make love.

For one thing, the ascent to orgasm (which, momentarily, involves extreme body tension) is much more dramatic if you first go *down* into a state of deep relaxation rather than starting from a state of semi-aroused agitation, says Martha Brown, a registered massage therapist in Charlottesville, Virginia.

"The biggest obstacle to great sex," Inkeles adds, "is stress." And sensual massage is one of the oldest and most reliable stress reducers in the world.

Massage, whether or not it's overtly sexual, is also just a delightful way to express affection. It's a way to explore the forgotten frontiers of your partner's body and in the process vastly expand your repertoire of touch. And it's a way of finding out what makes your lover feel good and what doesn't.

THE HOW-TO PART

Preparing for a sensuous massage is like setting the mood for love. It doesn't have to be terribly involved. Just find a space in your life where you're sure you won't be interrupted—the bedroom is fine. Take the phone off the hook. Lock the door. Put the clock in the drawer and forget about time. Don't focus on giving your lover a massage for any particular amount of time—just do it for as long as it feels good.

Massage oils are nice because they feel great and tend to make the skin more sensitive to touch. You can buy expensive massage oils, but ordinary safflower oil works fine, as does coconut oil. It's best to warm the oil a little before use. Try putting it in a plastic squeeze bottle for convenience. Instead of oil, some people like to use cornstarch, which is so silky to the touch that it almost feels wet.

Other things to remember:

■ People tend to touch each other during massage in the same way *they* like to be touched. The result: Men tend to massage women too firmly. The solution: Just keep asking for feedback. "How does this feel?" "Should I bear down harder?" "Is that too soft?" The only unforgivable sin of massage is to

• •

Stomach Punch and Judy

The quality of a man's marriage can influence his risk of getting an ulcer. In a five-year study of more than 8,000 subjects, researchers discovered that men who felt they got love and support from their wives were only half as likely to develop ulcers as men who felt they received no support.

make your partner feel uncomfortable. Says Inkeles: "One moment of pain destroys an hour of good massage."

■ People tend to hold lots of tension in their faces. Try massaging the forehead, jaw muscles, temples. Use strokes that smooth out or go across the lines on the face. Another great spot to focus on: the feet.

■ Women tend to hold tension in their neck and shoulders; men tend to hold it in the small of their backs, Inkeles says. Give those areas special attention.

■ Any spot where the skin is thin is especially sensitive, such as around the ankles, the insides of the arms and the neck.

You really don't need any fancy equipment to give a great massage, but sometimes a vibrator can be used for spice. Try strapping the device to the back of your hand, so your fingertips transmit the good vibrations.

MASSAGE AS THERAPY

The marvelously sensuous magic of massage has not been lost on sex therapists. In fact, a form of massage has been a key part of many sex therapy programs for the past 20 years. First developed by William Masters, M.D., and Virginia Johnson, of the Masters and Johnson Institute in St. Louis, sensate focus exercises, sometimes also called nondemand pleasuring, are a way for couples in sexual distress to break free of mutually reinforcing avoidance. But even people who are not having sex troubles can use them to great effect.

Basically, nondemand pleasuring works like this: A couple gets naked together in a quiet, romantic place and takes turns caressing each other's body. (Usually, at least to begin, the couple is seated, with the receiver sitting between the giver's legs.) There's just one rule: The breasts and genitals are off-limits, and so is intercourse. That way, there is no pressure to push forward to orgasm, no pressure to achieve anything or get anywhere, no pressure to return any favors. The only place to go is into the sensuality and stillness of the present moment.

—Stefan Bechtel

The Fine Art of Ogling

You spot her. You give her the once-over lightly.
You stare. She stares back. Now what?

• • • • • • • • • • • • • • • • • •

Ever notice how traveling through life is a little like vacationing in Boca Raton with Zsa Zsa Gabor? You sort of hate to say anything, but the plain truth, to pretzel-wrap a metaphor, is that Life overpacks, and it's you who ends up carrying the steamer crates filled with frilly little lessons and sequin-encrusted inescapable laws. Well, here's the deal. In this little space, at least, I'm your redcap. I guess sorting out the baggage is my job, given my profound affection not just for explanation but for pontification.

It's an easier job than most, owing to the plentiful supply of resources. In fact, the best part of life is the puzzle page, figuratively speaking, where enormously weighty subjects—death, women, work, government, shoes—can be discussed with proper deliberation. Here's something, for example: What does it mean when you're ogling a woman and she catches you at it and, instead of looking away, gives you a direct stare not once but *twice?*

I call this the Rule of Double Eye Contact on a Single Ogle. Case in point: two fortysomething guys. A mall. An escalator. Two women, mid-30s. One ogle. Two eye contacts.

The details: a sunny day, but brisk. Two friends—we'll call them Hoot and Gib—decide to meet for lunch at a downtown enclosed shopping mall. There's a quick dash into a Brooks Brothers outlet, where a suit is purchased within three minutes. Then there's lunch.

The dining area is one of those American adaptations of a Euro-trough, the standard street café. Next to the café is a descending escalator, and next to that is where our two chaps encamp for a bite. One guy, Hoot, is married, and he has his back to the escalator. He can't see anything, girl-wise. The other guy, Gib, is single, and he can see everything. The escalator practically dumps shoppers at his feet.

The conversation is a heavily fragmented one. Hoot talks about media coverage of the deficit. Gib is frequently distracted by the sudden appearance and descent of one or another metropolitan beauty. In the middle of a sentence, he suddenly clams up, raises one eyebrow in a sullen smolder and, frankly, ogles. He's been doing this for years, of course, and his scan is a well-practiced one. The face is his screening device. Bad face, back to the deficit. Good face, go directly to the shoes and work up. He ogles like a bibliophile, like a man who knows exactly which details and nuances create desirability and which ones are fatal flaws. Hoot waits patiently for the appraisal.

MEASURE YOURSELF

The Brown Corollary: A man ogles not just to fantasize about women but, according to writer Ian Brown, to see how he measures up as a man. Generally—and there are certainly exceptions to this corollary—he is making a precise calculation that involves this equation: Self-image divided by her beauty plus her availability equals relative worth of ogler. There are many tiny variables that can nudge the ultimate solution one way or another. For instance, you might look at a beautiful passerby and find she is almost certainly out of the range of your ability to attract women. Maybe the self-image part of the equation is too low or her beauty-plus-availability number is too high. But then you say to yourself "Sure, that's now. But a dash of Rogaine, a few years on carrots and sprouts and a Samsonite full of C-notes, and she'd be at my feet." Suddenly, your projected self-image numbers rise, and you find it more and more likely that not only could she be yours (if you really wanted) but maybe you wouldn't have time for her, what with all the other women around.

But back to the Double Eye Contact on a Single Ogle rule. When a normal guy is ogling, part of what he's actually doing is just thinking about what might politely be called a relationship. But sometimes in ogling, as in all relationships, things sort of sneak up on you. For instance, after a burger-and-fries' worth of idle ogling, Gib suddenly pales. "I got eye contact," he says tensely, almost grimly. "No, wait. That's it." His voice drops to a burdened whisper. "I got double eye contact."

The sequence is this: Contact. Ignition. Liftoff. Double eye contact in response to a single lingering ogle is a gesture of commitment more meaningful than many marriages. When a woman returns an ogle with a mere single glance, it can mean anything. Might mean: "What's he staring at? Is there toilet paper on my shoe?" Might mean: "Let's see what kind of jerk I'm dredging off the bottom of the gene pool today." Might mean: "Make a move, and I call the cops." Hence, most men disregard the Single Glance to an Ogle response.

I SEE YOU, TOO

A double glance, however, is something else. Double Eye Contact on a Single Ogle means this: "I know you're watching me, and I think you're sort of marginally interesting, and I think I'll see what you're made of, buster."

So. You ogle. She does a double take. Now what do you do? If you look away, too stunned or embarrassed to continue ogling, you're scrapple. A guy too cowardly to stand up for his own ogle isn't much of a man in most women's books. But if you continue to ogle in the face of a double glance, the ball's back in her court. If she looks away, no point. If she smiles, you can figure you've been asked to politely identify yourself, your motives, your marital standing. If your papers are in order, you get permission to cross the line, to go the next step. Whatever that is.

The Never-Fail Principle of Bad Timing: Women almost never return an ogle until your wife or girlfriend is looking—first at the woman, wondering who she's smiling at, and then at you when she figures it out.

Because we men ogle as a means of taking stock of ourselves, we know there's nothing intrinsically threatening about the whole activity. We don't ogle, after all, because we want to. We ogle because we have to. It's horrible sometimes. Call it ogle burden. But sometimes a man's gotta do what a man's gotta do.

TO EACH HIS OWN

That's why different men ogle in different ways. Involved men out with the objects of their involvement do an indirect ogle. They look around the supermarket as if they've never seen anything quite like it before. "Look at those lighting fixtures!" they seem to be saying. "And how about those metal shelving units!" Their necks are suddenly rubberized for such occasions, and the fact that a clearly ogleable woman just happens to be in line of sight is pure coincidence. That way, if the woman responds to the ogle with a smile, the guy can always look at his ferocious wife and shrug. Men know they can ogle their brains out and never get so much as a notice until one fine spring day when an ogling kind of guy and his principal sugar pie are out for a stroll. He tosses off an inconsequential ogle, and presto! He gets a double—no, a triple!—take in return. Then he starts explaining.

Guys out in packs do competitive ogling. A woman walks down the street, and there's a pack of wild oglers staring at her. She nervously glances over to make sure they aren't armed oglers, and instantly every man jack claims eye contact. "She was looking at me, man," one of them says, while the others produce documentary evidence refuting the claim.

A single-man ogle is a serious thing. Women know that. That may be why they so infrequently respond.

The Law of the Knowing Glance: The glance-to-ogle scenario has many variations. One of them involves the situation

• •

A Turn for the Worse

It's possible to injure your penis by bending it sharply during normal sexual intercourse. The damage can occur when the penis slips out during vigorous intercourse and then misses the vagina on the return thrust. Ouch! This can bring as much as 100 pounds of pressure to bear on the organ, much more than it was designed to withstand. "We've had patients coming to us saying they heard a snap, crackle, pop from their erections," says Irwin Goldstein, M.D., professor of urology at Boston University Medical Center. This forceful bending can damage the tissue and lining of the erection chamber. Dr. Goldstein estimates that as many as 15 percent of all cases of impotence are caused by injuries of this nature. Riskiest position: woman on top. (Forget all the stuff you saw in *Basic Instinct*.) If you suspect you've suffered this kind of injury, see a urologist. Four out of five cases can be treated successfully with medication.

reversed, where she is the ogler and you are the oglee. Women ogle as much as the next guy, by the way. Usually, they ogle other women, although since their mission in ogling is essentially fact gathering—"Why did she wear that scarf?" "You call that eyeshadow?" "Nice pumps"—it may be demeaning to ogling to call that ogling. Women sometimes ogle men. *That's* ogling. If you're on the receiving end, you might be well advised to invoke the Law of the Knowing Glance, which says an ogle is always trumped by a leer. In other words, you slowly look up and meet her gaze, while on your face you wear an expression that says "Was that good for you?"

NOW WHAT?

This has the effect of ram-injecting the encounter and giving it a NASA-level rate of acceleration. Suddenly, you're not just two strangers exchanging ogles for gapes. You're on intimate terms, with you, Mr. Mojo, in the driver's seat. You saw her ogle and raised her an innuendo. You can't lose. If she looks away, give her five minutes, and she'll ogle again. If she smiles, you can figure your glance was good enough that you can roll over and go to sleep. Either way, you'll have this encounter in the bag, if you'll pardon the play on words.

The Obviated Ogle Injunction: An ogle is diminished by overshadowing eccentricities. Let's say you're sitting alone in a subway car when a gaggle of art school painters' models—women who have been ogled with aesthetic passion—gets in. They're young, they're beautiful, and they stare right at you. The significance of their attention all depends on why they're staring. If it's because you're wearing a Santa suit and darning your socks, all ogles are off. No return glances are scored, and your self-image numbers are expressed in negatives.

Ogle-proof women: Finally, it's good to note that there are women who are at least ogle-resistant, if not downright ogle-proof. To wit: all nuns, the Queen of England, Andrea Dworkin and Imelda Marcos.

—Denis Boyles

Part 6

DISEASE-FREE LIVING

Home Remedies for Men

You need not run to the doctor for every ping and ding. Here are tips you can use to heal everyday health problems.

•••••••••••••••••••

IF IT'S NOT ONE THING, it's another. Hurt knees, backaches, bee stings, sore throats—minor injuries and health problems just seem to be a part of modern manhood. Sometimes you earn them: a black eye from an overexuberant pickup game, a burn suffered while trying to impress a new lover with your kitchen prowess. Other times trouble comes in less interesting packages: a wasp hiding in your sneaker, or a man with the flu sharing your cab.

Obviously, a serious illness or injury should receive proper medical attention. If your thumb is hanging by a thread from an altercation with a circular saw, you're beyond a little first-aid fix.

On the other hand, there are plenty of minor health bummers that you *can* treat yourself. Most of us have a basic understanding of over-the-counter medicines and first-aid procedures, a kind of primitive mental reference book of symptoms and their cures. (Sample entry: "Stomach hurts. Drink chalky stuff from bottle.") But there's more to self-care than chugging down store-bought remedies. Here's a look at some common ills and how you can put a stop to them. Bear in mind, though, that any problem that doesn't clear up or that gets worse with self-treatment should be taken to a doctor.

ATHLETE'S FOOT

"Athlete's foot" is a macho euphemism for what this rash really is: ringworm of the feet. Caused by a fungus that thrives in warm, moist conditions—like those in your shoes—it usually strikes the webbing between your fourth and fifth toes.

■ Rubbing or spraying antiperspirant on your feet can keep them from sweating and creating a fungus-friendly environment. You can use the same brand you use on your underarms, as long as it contains aluminum chloride, the active drying ingredient.

■ Before you spring for an expensive foot powder, try baking soda. Either sprinkle it on your feet and between your toes or make a paste by moistening one tablespoon of baking soda with lukewarm water. After about 15 minutes, rinse it off and dry thoroughly.

■ If you do opt for drugstore remedies such as Micatin or Tinactin, avoid creams, which can trap moisture in.

■ Help keep fungus away by disinfecting your shoes. Spray Lysol or another household disinfectant on a cloth and rub the inside of your shoes with it. Then blow air from a hair dryer into the shoe to help dry it out.

■ A mixture of two teaspoons of salt per pint of warm water provides a foot soak that zaps excess perspiration and hampers fungus growth, says Glenn Copeland, D.P.M., podiatrist for the Toronto Blue Jays. Soak your feet for five to ten minutes at a time, repeating often until the condition clears.

BACKACHE

It doesn't take rocket science to treat lower back pain effectively, says Brent V. Lovejoy, D.O., an occupational medicine specialist in Denver and a consultant to the construction industry. Seventy to 90 percent of back pain goes away by itself or with some minor home treatment. Rest and drugstore pain relievers are what most doctors recommend *initially* for a sudden attack of back pain. You shouldn't need more than two or three days' bed rest, however. A study at the University of Washington School of Medicine found that back pain sufferers who were advised to stay in bed just two days missed 45 percent fewer days of work during the following three months than patients advised to rest for a full week. Muscles may weaken quickly with bed rest, and weak muscles can perpetuate an aching back. See a doctor if your back pain doesn't improve after three days—or if the pain is so bad that you can't budge from the bed.

■ You may be able to soothe the ache by icing your back. Lie on your stomach with a towel on your back, and have someone massage your aching spots with the ice. (The ice should not be applied directly to the skin.) You can also lie down on your back with your knees bent and slide a bag of crushed ice (wrapped in a wet towel) under the sore spot.

■ Try this relaxation tactic: Lie flat on your back on the floor, with your knees bent at a 90-degree angle and your calves resting on the seat of a chair. This position helps relieve pressure on your back.

■ It's also possible to relieve pain with an acupressure treatment using a tennis ball. Lie on a hard surface and position the tennis ball under you so that it is pressing against a tender spot. Roll onto the ball gradually, utilizing your body weight until the pain and tenderness subside.

■ One study found that 80 percent of back pain sufferers reported rapid and significant relief when they switched from basic street shoes to lightweight, flexible-soled shoes with shock-absorbing cushions.

BLACK EYES AND BRUISES

The worst thing about a black eye is putting up with the inevitable questions about how you got it, especially if your shiner came not from defending your honor but from walking into a door.

■ The first course of treatment for all bruises is ice, which constricts blood vessels so that less blood spills into the tissues around the injury. Apply an ice pack wrapped in a towel for about 15 minutes, then allow the skin to "warm" naturally for about 10 minutes before you put on the ice pack again.

■ The day *after* applying ice packs, switch to heat to dilate blood vessels and improve circulation. A heating pad or a warm, wet washcloth will help.

■ If you want a pain reliever, avoid aspirin. It's an anticoagulant, which means it prevents the blood from clotting and can lead to a bigger bruise. Stick with Tylenol and other acetaminophen products.

■ If you bruise easily, eat more foods high in vitamin C, such as broccoli and citrus fruits. Studies show that vitamin C helps build skin tissue.

COLDS AND FLU

Your average cold or flu can be downright painful if it hits you the wrong way—some people have earaches so bad that they wonder if Van Gogh wasn't just a sane, talented guy with blocked eustachian tubes. There are, however, some less permanent treatments for these and other cold-related aches.

Earaches can knock you flat on your back, but to get relief, try sitting upright for a few minutes, recommends Hueston King, M.D., of the University of Texas Southwestern Medical Center at Dallas. Elevating your head may help your ears start draining. Other solutions:

■ Turn on C-Span. A good yawn will flex the muscle that opens clogged eustachian tubes, the ducts that connect the ear to the back of the throat.

■ Using eardrops or a few drops of white vinegar can be an effective treatment for an outer-ear infection. Drops are useless for a middle-ear infection, which is closed off from the outer ear. How do you tell what kind of infection you have? Grab your ear, pull it forward gently, and wiggle it. If it hurts like crazy, you probably have an outer-ear problem and can use the drops. If it doesn't hurt, you've probably got a middle-ear infection, which calls for decongestants, says Dr. King.

■ The popular home remedy of resting the ear against a hot water bottle can actually make the pain worse by causing the blood vessels to swell. Instead, use an ice pack (wrapped in a towel) to help reduce swelling and get the ear cavity to open.

Use a decongestant to help open *clogged sinus passages.* Be careful with medicated nasal sprays—they can be highly addictive. "There's never a week that goes by that I don't have to pull someone off an addiction," Dr. King says, although he admits that for emergencies, these sprays can safely be used for a day or two. Saline sprays, available at drugstores without a prescription, are safer alternatives.

If you're battling *hoarseness,* you can impress your friends with your Bill Clinton impersonation, or you can help relieve your symptoms by breathing moistened air from a humidifier or vaporizer. And of course, drink lots of liquids—peach or apricot nectar will provide vitamin C without the acidity of orange juice, which can irritate a sore throat. (More tips for coping with sore throat are listed below.)

HEADACHES

Headaches can generally be classified into three categories: tension headaches, migraines and sinus headaches.

Tension headaches make up 75 to 80 percent of all headaches. It's believed they come about when a tense muscle group—usually in the scalp, neck, shoulders or back—bears down on the blood vessels leading to the head.

Aspirin, acetaminophen and ibuprofen are all fine remedies, but there are other, nonmedicinal ways of relieving the pain.

■ For a mild tension headache, try taking a walk. Some experts think that easy exercise can ease headache pain by releasing endorphins, the body's own pain-killing chemicals, while others theorize that it's simply the relaxing effects of a light workout that help.

■ If you can't get away from your desk, try this simple tension reliever: Place your thumb or index finger on one of the two prominent bony areas on your temple, closest to the pain point. Firmly rub in small circles, directing the pressure against the bone. Keep it up for about two minutes.

■ Compresses can also help lessen severe tension headaches, but whether to use cold or heat is an individual matter. Try a cold pack against the back of your neck first. If that fails to bring relief after 20 minutes, switch to a hot compress.

Migraine pain comes from the swelling of blood vessels in the brain, often brought about by changes in weather, altitude or sleep patterns as well as by light and motion.

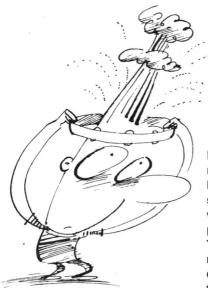

Relief Is at Band

For people who suffer from migraines, relief may be at hand—or at head. In a recent study, a special headband was able to ease migraine pain 87 percent of the time. The elastic headband contains moveable rubber disks designed to put pressure on the location of maximum pain.

■ For migraines, aspirin and ibuprofen are the best nonprescription pain relievers because they help reduce swelling. Aspirin products that contain caffeine may be even more effective, since caffeine constricts blood vessels. Taking aspirin regularly—even when you don't have a migraine—may keep migraines at bay. In one study, men who took one regular adult aspirin tablet every other day reported 20 percent fewer migraines than those taking a sugar pill.

■ You may also want to ask your doctor about Imitrex, a new drug that constricts the specific blood vessels in the head and neck that cause migraines. Currently up for approval by the Food and Drug Administration, it may be available soon.

■ Those seeking drug-free pain relief should bypass the medicine cabinet and head for the bedroom. Researchers at Southern Illinois University School of Medicine reported that up to half of the migraine sufferers they studied found some relief from their symptoms after sex. Although there's no evidence the cure works for men (only women participated in the study), "I've got a migraine" might prove to be the best sympathy line since "They're shipping me off to Parris Island tomorrow."

■ Chronic (or just less romantic) migraine sufferers may want to consult their doctors about using a portable oxygen tank. Pure oxygen breathed for 10 to 30 minutes may halt migraine pain by reducing blood flow to the brain.

Sinus headaches can be relieved by applying cold packs to the forehead and those sinuses hiding directly below your eyes and just above your teeth. An over-the-counter decongestant will help relieve sinus pain, but avoid decongestants that include antihistamines. They dry up your nose and thicken mucus—exactly what you don't want.

HEEL SPURS

Heel spurs are bony protrusions on the bottom of the feet, caused by continuous pulling of the ligament that runs across the sole. Runners and others who are hard on their feet are susceptible to them.

■ When your heel spur is acting up, try applying an ice pack wrapped in a towel to stop the pain. Keep your heel under ice for ten minutes, then remove the pack for another ten minutes.

■ Don't walk around barefoot, says William Van Pelt, D.P.M., a podiatrist in Houston and former president of the American Academy of Podiatric Sports Medicine. "Walking barefoot stretches out the ligament on the bottom of the foot even further."

■ Over-the-counter arch supports and heel cups, which are sold in most drugstores and sporting goods stores, help those with heel spurs in two ways: "They support the arch, which controls excess foot rolling or movement, and they help elevate the heel a bit, which takes some of the pressure off the spur," says Dr. Van Pelt.

INSECT BITES

Although insect bites rarely require medical attention, they are bothersome. You may like the idea of squashing the perpetrator, but you'll feel even better if you can squash the pain.

■ Rubbing on a meat tenderizer containing papain can take the ouch out of that bite: Make a paste with water and the meat tenderizer, and apply it directly on the bite area as soon as possible. For severe itching and swelling, apply some calamine lotion.

■ Other remedies in your house include a paste made by mixing table salt with water and applying it to the bite. Another way: Place ice packs wrapped in towels on the area for 10 minutes. Or dissolve one teaspoon of baking soda in a glass of water, dip a cloth into the solution, and place it on the bite for 20 minutes.

■ If you're outdoors, pack the bite with mud, suggests Rodney Basler, M.D., a dermatologist in Fremont, Nebraska, and an assistant professor of internal medicine at the University of Nebraska Medical Center in Omaha. "I'm not sure *why* it works, but it works."

JOINT PAIN

Your knees and your shoulders are the most used joints in your body—and are commonly abused and injured.

■ Use ibuprofen to calm inflammation and soreness, but when you resume your activity, try to do it when you're not taking the medicine, so you can feel the pain if your joints send out warning signals.

■ Another pain reliever you can try is bromelain. Made from pineapple, bromelain is touted as a natural anti-inflammatory that is thought to speed healing. It is sold in tablet form in some health-food stores. A word of caution, though: Bromelain can cause a rash in some people, so stop taking it if your skin starts to feel itchy.

■ Applying ice will help force your body to flush the joint with blood and oxygen, elements vital for repair. Apply ice wrapped in a towel to the sore joint for no longer than 20 minutes every hour.

■ Shoulder pain frequently results from repetitive motion, whether it's caused by your job or by playing sports. To remedy this problem and help prevent it in the future, perform full range-of-motion stretching. For instance, if you have shoulder pain after playing tennis, perform some gentle stretching exercises such as rotating your arm inward and outward and doing slow, full arm circles in both directions.

■ When it comes to preventing knee trouble, look into your sole. Place the shoes you exercise in on a table at eye level to see whether the shoes stand straight up. If the soles have worn down unevenly, the shoes will tip out or in—and tip you off that it's time for a new pair. Also examine around the midsole and sides to spot excessive wear. Many shoes will begin to severely break down after 300 miles.

■ If joint pain is severe or there is swelling or weakness, especially in the knee, be sure to see your doctor for a more thorough examination. Swelling could be a sign of internal knee damage.

NAUSEA

Next time you feel like George Bush at a sushi bar, try these quick remedies to quell your queasy stomach.

■ Whip up a Maalox cocktail. Put a few drops of spirits of peppermint in your Maalox and mix it with one quart of distilled water. Take a few sips of this to soothe your upset stomach and use the rest later, as needed.

■ A few slugs of soft drink that's gone flat can help settle your stomach. Or look for the flat syrup of Coca-Cola, available in some drugstores, and sip it over cracked ice.

■ Some people find relief from nausea—especially the kind that comes from motion sickness—by applying pressure to the inside of the wrist near the center. Sea Bands, special wristbands that put pressure on the inside wrist area, were created for seasickness but are now used for other types of nausea. They can be found at boat dealers, in some sporting goods stores and in most local American Automobile Association offices.

■ Don't forget Dramamine. Although little is known about how Dramamine works to ease nausea, and not everyone responds to it, you can give it a try and keep this over-the-counter medication on hand if it works for you.

OVERWORKED MUSCLES

So you got suckered into helping a buddy move across town? Ease the next-day soreness with these tactics.

■ If you're feeling courageous, try the hot-and-cold-shower remedy. Take a hot shower for two minutes. Then turn on the cold and let it run full throttle for 30 seconds. Repeat the process five to ten times. As you switch from hot water to cold, your blood vessels actually widen and narrow, flushing lactic acid—which causes muscle soreness—out of the muscles.

■ At the University of Colorado, the Buffaloes football team has its own secret weapon for combating muscle soreness: massage. Following games and after the Buffaloes' toughest workouts, players are given body massages to help move along waste products such as lactic acid that build up during exercise. Massage helps push the acid out of the muscle, helping recovery time.

RASHES AND HIVES

The best all-around Rx for breakouts is a little R and R. When you're under stress, your body releases chemicals that force white blood cells to clog blood vessel walls beneath the skin. That reaction causes redness and irritation on the skin surface and exacerbates your breakout. So stop worrying and take action.

■ Applying a lotion of crushed vitamin C tablets and water directly on skin may cure many rashes because of the vitamin's ability to neutralize free radicals. (No, not your activist friends from your college days; these are oxygen molecules that occur naturally in the body and appear to have a damaging effect on body tissues.)

■ Try dabbing on calamine lotion or alcohol to soothe your itching, or apply a cold compress over hives to help shrink blood vessels.

■ Take an over-the-counter antihistamine such as Benadryl or Chlor-Trimeton to halt the release of hive-causing histamines.

SORE THROAT

Flu season may be over, but you can get a sore throat for a lot of other reasons—from viral or bacterial infections, dry air, exposure to cigarette smoke and other irritants or too much cheering at a Red Sox game.

■ Pop a zinc gluconate tablet. In one study at the Clayton Foundation Biochemical Institute at the University of Texas at Austin, zinc proved to be an effective reliever of throat soreness and some other cold symptoms. The trick to this home remedy is to let the dissolved zinc bathe your throat for a while; don't just swallow the tablet. The lozenges should be used for no more than seven days, because large amounts of zinc can interfere with your body's ability to absorb other minerals.

■ Another idea is to do as the Romans do. "When a sore throat is caused by a virus infection, as opposed to bacteria, eating garlic can bring quicker relief," suggests Yu-Yan Yeh, Ph.D., associate professor of nutrition at Pennsylvania State University. "Garlic has been shown to have antiviral and antifungal activities." You may want to try an eye-opening cocktail of tomato or mixed vegetable juice, two garlic cloves and a dash of Worcestershire sauce. Run it through a blender and drink.

■ Use lozenges containing menthol or eucalyptus, benzocaine or phenol.

■ Breathe through your nose and keep your mouth shut to help keep your throat from getting dry.

■ Gargling with warm salt water will also help.

■ A cold pack (many drugstores sell ice collars) will help reduce swelling in the throat as well.

SPRAINS AND STRAINS

Knowing the difference between a sprain and a strain makes all the difference when it comes to treatment.

Sprains occur because of excessive stretching or tearing of a ligament, one of those tough bands of elastic-like tissue attached to a joint. You'll feel pain for sure, but there's usually another sign as well: The area may be swollen and black and blue.

■ Most experts recommend immediate icing for sprains. The cold deadens the pain and decreases blood flow, which

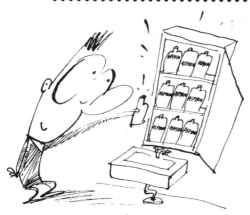

Hi-Fiber Aspirin

We've all heard that eating a diet rich in citrus fruits, vegetables and high-fiber grains such as bran and whole wheat can help prevent colon cancer. Now new research suggests that regular use of aspirin makes the benefits of a high-fiber diet even stronger. The long-term study found that men who regularly ate the most vegetables and fiber and took aspirin 16 or more times per month were 2.4 times less likely to die of colon cancer than those who ate few vegetables or fiber—and took no aspirin.

lessens swelling. Apply the ice (wrapped in a towel) for 15 to 20 minutes, then take it off for an equal period of time, four or five times daily for at least two days.

■ After treating it with ice, elevate the sprained joint above heart level.

Strains occur when a muscle is stretched or partially torn. If you have a strain, you can tell because it won't get swollen or black and blue like a sprain. And the treatment is different.

■ Heat works better for strains because it increases blood flow and the influx of oxygen to muscles, which speeds production of skin tissue, a crucial step in the healing process. Just put a hot water bottle or heating pad on the affected area for 15 to 30 minutes, four to six times a day.

■ Don't rub on Ben-Gay or another ointment before applying heat; the skin can absorb so much of the cream that it can cause deep blistering.

SWIMMER'S EAR

Everyone has bacteria in his ear canals (yes, even Cindy Crawford). When the ear canal gets waterlogged and irritated, these bacteria start to multiply, and the result is a stuffed-up, itchy ear that feels swollen and tender.

■ Dry up the bacteria's soggy homestead by draining and drying your ears after swimming. Lean over sideways, and pull your ear to straighten the canal and let water drain out.

■ If swimmer's ear is a recurrent problem for you, you can find relief either in your local drugstore, from antiseptic eardrops such as Auro-Dri and Swim Ear, or in your kitchen pantry. Get an eyedropper-style bottle from the pharmacy and fill it with a mixture of half white vinegar and half rubbing alcohol. Tilt your head and put in enough drops to fill the ear canal. Then tilt your head the other way to let the solution pour out. Growth of bacteria is inhibited in this acidic environment.

■ Next time you head to the pool, try using silicone putty earplugs to help protect infection-prone ears. Make a ball of silicone bigger than the entrance to the ear canal and mush it so that it covers the opening but does not go deep inside. Don't use hard plugs, which can abrade the skin and *cause* infection.

TENNIS ELBOW

Whether you stroke a tennis ball or tote a briefcase, *any* strain of the forearm tendons can make your elbow sore. Here are some hints from the masters of arms.

▪ First, rest your arm. If swelling and soreness have already set in, your elbow needs at least three weeks' respite from playing tennis, says Susan Perry, a physical therapist specializing in sports medicine at the Fort Lauderdale Sports Medicine Center in Fort Lauderdale, Florida.

▪ While you're resting it, soothe that sore elbow by rubbing it with ice wrapped in a towel.

▪ Zap elbow pain with a topical over-the-counter ointment called Zostrix. Made from a derivative of hot peppers, it works as a temporary anesthetic.

▪ Using a cheap metal racket or an old wooden one? If you've got tennis elbow, you're better off switching to a lighter racket made from a graphite compound. The heavier metal or wooden frame puts more strain on your arm.

TOOTHACHE

It's not only Riddick Bowe's sparring partners who have to deal with mouth pain. Knowing what to do for occasional soreness will help you keep your chin up.

Toothaches that last more than several minutes or that come on without provocation warrant a visit to the dentist, says Thomas Lundeen, D.M.D., codirector of the University of North Carolina Clinical Pain Program. But if you can't get an emergency appointment, there are some things you can do to ease your agony until you can get to the chair.

▪ Hot, moist towels applied to your jaw over the pain may help.

▪ If the pain gets only worse with heat, try cold packs on the jaw for 15 to 20 minutes, four or five times a day.

▪ Dr. Lundeen recommends over-the-counter toothache drops containing oil of cloves (eugenol) for temporary relief.

▪Aspirin and ibuprofen are also good for temporary relief.

But if there's redness or swelling around the tooth, or if you feel sick or feverish, see your dentist fast.

—Sid Kirchheimer and Jeff Stevenson

Your Prostate Is Calling

When nature calls too often, it could be that your prostate is trying to send you a message.

● ● ● ● ● ● ● ● ● ● ● ● ● ● ● ● ● ● ●

IT'S THE MIDDLE OF THE NIGHT, and that silent alarm clock in your bladder awakens you for a trip to the bathroom. Funny, you seem to be visiting the men's room at work more often, too, never leaving with the feeling that you've completely finished what you went to do.

The source of this little problem just might be your prostate, a small gland that happens to be wrapped around the urethra (urinary exit pipe) and that most men don't even notice until they're between 40 and 50 years of age. The prostate's job in life is to secrete the fluid and enzyme mixture that sperm require for good health and upward mobility. Then at middle age, the gland typically begins to swell. In some cases, it can grow to the size of an orange, which has the effect of strangling the urethra. Doctors call the condition benign prostatic hyperplasia (BPH). Early symptoms include frequent urination, trouble starting the flow, weak flow and a feeling that even when you're done, you're not quite done.

Don't be alarmed if you've got some of these problems. The "benign" in *BPH* means it isn't cancerous. But you still want to deal with it as soon as you can. In advanced cases, an enlarged prostate can completely block the flow of urine. If you wait that long, you're going to need surgery, best described as a Roto-Rooter job in which the surgeon shaves away the portion of the prostate that's pressing on the urethra. It is painful and unpleasant and takes a few months to fully recover from.

Why does the prostate grow? "Good question. We don't really know," says Robert P. Huben, M.D., chief of urologic oncology at Roswell Park Cancer Institute in Buffalo. Dr. Huben and other experts believe the gland's tendency to swell may have something to do with the male hormone testosterone. Eunuchs don't get BPH. For the rest of the male population, however, the condition is very common. In fact, it affects as many as 60 percent of men over age 50 and 15 percent over age 40. (See the self-test on the opposite page to measure how you're doing, prostate-wise.)

Perhaps because the condition is so prevalent and creeps up so slowly, many middle-aged men don't realize that something's wrong. They figure it is an inevitable change that they have no control over. But the fact is, particularly in the early stages of BPH, there's much you can do to improve. Here are the best tips for reducing symptoms of prostate trouble.

Don't hold it in. If you need to urinate frequently, logic may tell you to train your bladder by waiting as long as you can. Logic has been wrong before, and it's wrong here. "You may actually harm yourself by waiting too long," says Patrick Walsh, M.D., chairman of urology at Johns Hopkins University. "When urine backs up too far, it can damage the kidneys." Better to urinate as soon as you feel the need.

Ejaculate regularly. Tough medicine, we know. But doing so may keep prostatic ducts from getting clogged and backed up. "It can only help," says Kenneth Goldberg, M.D., founder and director of the Male Health Center in Dallas.

Don't drink too much. Avoid all liquids after 6:00 or 7:00 P.M. if your sleep has been interrupted frequently (say, two or more times a night) by the urge to pee. Especially don't drink alcohol, a central nervous system depressant that reduces muscle tone throughout the body, including in the bladder, causing it to retain urine. Day or night, limit drinks containing caffeine. These make you urinate more and increase stress on the bladder, causing it to feel full even when it isn't.

Limit spicy foods. Like alcohol, spicy foods may increase bladder irritability.

Eat more vegetables. Male hormone levels drop on a vegetarian diet, and that may explain why, for example, BPH is rarer in certain Asian cultures that are largely vegetarian.

Lower your cholesterol. Cholesterol is converted to male hormone in the body. It's been observed that enlarged prostate tissue is very high in cholesterol. Some doctors claim an improvement in symptoms, if not in prostate size,

● ●

FLOW CHART

To see if you are experiencing signs of prostate trouble, answer the following questions. Over the past month, how often have you . . .

1. Had a sensation of not emptying your bladder completely after you finished urinating?

0   1   2   3   4   5

2. Had to urinate again less than two hours after urinating?

0   1   2   3   4   5

3. Found that the flow of urine stopped and started several times?

0   1   2   3   4   5

4. Found it difficult to postpone urination?

0   1   2   3   4   5

5. Had a weak urine stream?

0   1   2   3   4   5

6. Had to push or strain to begin urination?

0   1   2   3   4   5

7. Had to get up to urinate after going to bed, on a typical night?

0   1   2   3   4   5

Add up your score: _____

If you scored 10 or more, visit a urologist for an examination. *Note:* This is not a test for prostate cancer. Ask your doctor about prostate exams and screening for prostate cancer.

Test courtesy of the Male Health Center, Dallas, Texas.

● ●

by getting their patients to lower cholesterol.

Get enough zinc. Concentrations of zinc tend to be low in men with prostate disease—hence the thinking that increasing zinc intake to normal levels may help. Foods that are rich in zinc include oysters and herring. Oatmeal, wheat bran, milk, peas and nuts also contain the mineral.

Don't sit for too long. That's your prostate you're sitting on all day. Get up regularly and walk around.

Get some exercise. No, there's no prostate-specific workout. Rather, many physicians have observed that men in good shape, with good body tone, are less likely to have prostate trouble than sedentary men are.

If your symptoms are more severe, and none of the above methods provides adequate relief, two medications can help. The first of these is Hytrin, which relaxes the nerve endings of the bladder neck and prostate to de-stress muscles in the region. James H. Gilbaugh, Jr., M.D., clinical instructor in urology at Oregon Health Sciences University, reports that one-third to one-half of BPH patients treated with Hytrin get some relief with this method. The Food and Drug Administration's approval for Hytrin's use in treating BPH is pending.

The other drug is Proscar, much ballyhooed as the first nonsurgical way to actually shrink the prostate gland. In the past, the trouble with a drug approach has been that you can't block testosterone without affecting potency. Proscar works by reducing a hormone related to testosterone that is specifically responsible for prostate enlargement. There is no effect on testosterone levels body-wide, and side effects are rare. A recent study of 895 men with BPH, reported in the *New England Journal of Medicine,* found that the drug reduced the size of the prostate by about 20 percent on average, enough to boost urine flow by 23 percent. Potency problems were reported in about 5 percent.

Because these two drugs act in different ways, there are currently several studies under way to see if using them in combination would be better than using them separately. Though the results aren't yet available, many doctors are already prescribing both, hoping for a one-two punch.

—Steven Slon

Breathe Easy

*How to nip allergies in the bud when
there's something in the air.*

●●●●●●●●●●●●●●●●●●●

Aʜ, SPRINGTIME. Children frolicking. Flowers blooming.
Backyard birds shoving writhing larvae down the throats of
their young. It's days like these that you want to get outside
and take a run through the cool, fresh air.

But instead, you're laid up on the couch with a box of
Kleenex and a bottle of pills you picked up down at the Stop 'n'
Pop pharmacy, suffering through your latest attack of hay fever.

If it seems that your allergies have been a lot worse over
the past few years, you're probably right. And if it seems that
everyone you know is having the same trouble, you're probably right again. "There has been an increase in allergies right
across the board," says William Davis, M.D., of the Columbia
University College of Physicians and Surgeons. One of the
main reasons has been increasingly intense allergy seasons,
particularly on the East Coast and especially in springtime.
The combination of mild winters, increased rainfall and cool
springs leads to a concentrated pollen season in May and
June. Add to that the increased popularity of home humidi-
fiers, which can promote the growth of allergy-triggering
dust mites, and enough air pollution to get Al Gore within
sneezing range of the White House, and you've got a strange
brew swirling through the winds.

Your age is a factor, too. "A lot of people who had allergies when they were kids were told 'You'll grow out of them,'
and you know what? They did," says William Storms, M.D.,
associate clinical professor of medicine at the University of
Colorado School of Medicine. "But when people hit 30, 35,
40, their allergies tend to come back, though we don't know
why. I see a lot of people who come in and say 'I've never
had an allergy in my life.' Then when you talk to them, they
remember that when they were kids, they were going to the
doctor a lot, or they had a lot of earaches. It was allergies;
they just never knew."

TAKE COMFORT

You could take comfort in the fact that a lot of other people are sniffling right along with you. In fact, it happens that President Bill Clinton is allergic to dust, pollen, mold spores, cat dander and a host of other things. Watching him struggle with Washington's allergy season may provide you with a little companionship. On the other hand, you've got your own problems: Softball league is starting soon, the kids are complaining because you're always laid up on the couch, and Jenkins in accounting is outmaneuvering you for a promotion. You need to start feeling healthy *now*.

The good news is that there are steps you can take today that will help you overcome your allergy attacks and get back on the playing field, regardless of how high the grass is. But first, you've got to understand your opponent. An allergy is basically a case of mistaken identity.

Because of the particular chemistry that occurred when your mom met your dad, you were born with an immune system that identified one or more harmless substances, such as ragweed pollen, as a threat and produced antibodies to them. Now whenever you come in contact with these airborne Barney Fifes, your body reacts as though a legion of Dirty Harrys has invaded. The antibodics stimulate specialized cells in the nose, eyes, skin and respiratory system to release a number of substances, among them histamine. It is histamine that causes the sneezing, watery eyes and sinus congestion or, in the skin, inflammation, itching and rashes.

HAY FEVER

Although you can be allergic to almost everything, from your pet guinea pig to your mother-in-law, the most common causes of "hay fever" symptoms are dust (or, more accurately, the microscopic mites that call it home), pollen (from trees, weeds and grasses), mold spores and animal dander (especially from cats). All these allergens can elicit many of the same symptoms as your run-of-the-mill cold, but there are factors that distinguish an allergic reaction from a viral infection.

Ever get a cold that simply wouldn't go away, or one that seemed to come back every year at the same time? That's an allergy, pal. But how do you know for sure that it's an allergy and not the flu? Both can give you a runny, stuffy nose, but a cold or flu will produce a thick, sticky mucus (sorry, it's our job to talk about this stuff) and an occasional sneeze, while an allergy will elicit a thin, watery discharge and a series of prolonged bouts of sneezing. You may also itch on your nose, ears and scalp and between the shoulder blades.

With an allergy, you'll also be missing the fever and achiness that often accompany a virus, and your eyes will likely be itchy. But most significantly, your symptoms won't go away in a week, like cold and flu symptoms do. If you've been laid up more than seven days, think allergy.

So now you know what allergies are. The real question is, what can you do about them? First, you've got to know exactly what it is you're allergic to. Sometimes this is no more difficult than noticing when your allergies act up. If your nose starts twitching whenever your girlfriend's cat climbs on your lap, you've probably figured out that heavy petting is a no-no. But other allergies are harder to track down. Is there a particular time of year that starts you sneezing? Trees such as ash, birch, cedar, elm, maple and oak pollinate in the early spring, beginning in January in the south and March in the north. Ragweed, the most common allergen, pollinates at the end of the summer. If your sneezing and wheezing is a year-round problem or is most notable in winter, when you spend most of your time indoors, you may be allergic to dust. If you start to sneeze when you're cleaning a damp basement or raking leaves, it might be mold that's inciting your system to riot.

It's not always possible to figure this out by yourself, since frequently you're allergic not to one substance but to a variety of things. Consult an allergist for a skin test, in which pinpricks are made on the skin and then exposed to the most common allergens to see which cause a mild inflammation. This is preferable to the more expensive blood test, in which a sample of your blood is extracted and sent to a lab for testing. "The skin test is still the gold standard," says Dr. Davis.

The allergist may then suggest a variety of medications. We'll discuss that option farther down, but there are a number of steps you can take to manage and control your allergies that just might save you a trip to the drugstore.

● ●

INSECT ASIDE

We've all been stung by the occasional bee or wasp, and for most of us, the incident resulted in some intense but brief pain and a few naughty words. But a small percentage of men react with severe symptoms, the most extreme of which is anaphylactic shock, a sometimes fatal reaction marked by bronchial spasms, plummeting blood pressure and irregular heartbeat. "A large number of 'golf course coronaries' may actually be fatal insect stings that go unrecognized," says Bob Lanier, M.D, an allergist in Fort Worth, Texas. He points out that while most people who have insect allergies are aware of them, others may acquire the allergy over time, slowly developing increasingly severe symptoms that are never recognized. Here are some warning signs to look out for.

■ An exaggerated reaction at the site of the sting (such as intense pain, severe swelling or itching), especially if it continues for more than 72 hours

■ A reaction away from the sting, such as breaking out in hives

■ Tightness in the chest, wheezing or faintness

If you have any of these symptoms, consult a doctor immediately. Since you may be at risk for an even more severe reaction in the future, your doctor will likely administer an allergy test, and if it's positive, he may equip you with a first-aid kit to carry with you. It generally consists of a syringe containing epinephrine, a hormone that relaxes bronchial muscles and jump-starts the heart. For those who can't stand sticking themselves, spring-action auto-injectors are also available. Ask your doctor about them.

● ●

DUST

Suck it up. Maybe vacuuming is not too high on your priority list (somewhere between returning your neighbor's power shears and alphabetizing your collection of Barry Manilow records). But if you're allergic to dust, you're paying a price for your slovenly ways. While a conventional vacuum can allow dust to escape back into the air, outfitting it with a high-efficiency dust bag will help cut down your exposure. Filteraire bags from Eureka (800-282-2886) and Micro-Fresh bags from Royal Appliance (800-321-1134) use electrostatically charged fibers to trap microscopic particles of dust, pollen and bacteria. Fresh Aire bags from Sears Brand Central do the same for Kenmore canister vacuums. If you really want to get serious, invest in a Nilfisk allergy vacuum, which comes equipped with a powerful HEPA (high-efficiency particle accumulation) filter to trap dust mite particles. To locate a dealer near you, contact Nilfisk of America (800-241-9420).

Catch the dust. Consider using a HEPA air cleaner such as the Enviracaire (800-332-1110). This is a lightweight, portable appliance that can clean the air in a room up to six times an hour.

Don't be a carpet crawler. Dust mites love carpeting, so consider area rugs, or no rugs, instead of wall-to-wall. If it's not possible to switch, you can purchase Acarosan, a mite-killing powder, at some pharmacies or through Fisons Pharmaceuticals Corporation (800-999-6483). Brush it into the carpet, wait 12 hours, then vacuum. Acarosan has been shown to keep carpets mite-free for up to six months.

Try synthetic sleep. Wrapping your mattress in plastic will keep dust down while you sleep. For a more comfortable night, you might prefer Allergy Control covers, which have a dust mite–blocking barrier on one side and a soft, outer layer made from cotton-blend fabric. Contact Allergy Control Products (800-422-3878). Also, try sleeping on pillows with synthetic stuffing (such as Hollofil or Dacron), which can be laundered. Washing them in hot water will help you smite the mites. A Vellux blanket, made from insulating nylon fabric, can also be washed repeatedly in hot water and will stand up better than wool or down. For ordering information, contact West Point Pepperell (800-533-8229).

Keep your ego off the shelf. Unless you have a maid, put all those high-school trophies, autographed baseballs, pictures of your car and other knickknacks away—they can collect dust. If you can't live without looking at your *tchotchkes,* get yourself a trophy case and shut it.

. . . .

PRIME SUSPECTS

Know your enemy and how to fight it.

Allergen	Source	Season	Solutions
Dust mites	Dust, especially from carpeting and upholstery	Year-round	Use a dehumidifier in most-used rooms. Get rid of extra carpeting, upholstery and blankets. Use plastic or dust-proof covering on mattresses and pillows.
Pollen	Trees, grasses and weeds	Spring, summer and autumn	Cut back on outdoor activities before 10:00 A.M. Air-condition home and car. Hire someone to tend your lawn. Avoid exercising on windy days or near vacant lots. Wear glasses or sunglasses out-

. . . .

POLLEN

Don't hang around. Trying to save money by hanging your clothes on a line to dry can wind up costing you in allergy medication. Air-dried clothes can pick up pollen.

Use a conditioner. Air-conditioning helps filter out pollen and other airborne irritants from outdoors. Have your

Allergen	Source	Season	Solutions
			doors. Shower after any outdoor activities.
Mold spores	Damp bathrooms and basements; grass clippings and leaves	Year-round	Use a shower fan in the bathroom and a dehumidifier in other rooms. Avoid going out after a rainfall, when mold spores prosper. Hire someone to rake leaves for you. Fix any leaky fixtures.
Pet dander	Household pets	Year-round	Keep pets out of your bedroom. Consult your veterinarian for an anti-allergenic pet shampoo. Wash hands after handling animals.

air conditioner cleaned regularly to prevent mold growth. Clean the filter and water pan periodically for the same reason.

Visit nice places, but don't live there. Mountain and desert climes have lower pollen counts, and taking a vacation during your allergy season is a good way to cut down on your exposure. But a vacation haven can be a better place to visit than to live. Many people actually move in an attempt to outrun their allergies, but a few years down the road, they usually find something blooming in their new hometown that sets their nose twitching.

Landscape smartly. You might have a fondness for juniper trees, but if you fill your lawn with them, the constant exposure could make you sensitive to their pollen. The best bet is a mix of trees, says botanist James Thompson, Ph.D. "If you go for diversity, the plants will pollinate at different times, and with just one plant pollinating, you might not become sensitized," he says. If you insist on symmetry, opt for pine trees, which generally have the lowest incidence of allergies.

Shower often. "Pollen is magnetically attracted to hair," says Dr. Thompson. If you've spent some time outdoors during allergy season, change your clothes and shower as soon as you come inside.

Be a foul-weather friend. Rain tends to wash pollen out of the air, so exercising after a rainfall is a good way to enjoy the great outdoors if you're pollen-sensitive. On the other hand, if you are allergic to molds, it's not a good idea. Mold spore counts, which are ten times higher than pollen counts in most parts of the country, can soar even higher after a rain, exceeding 10,000 spores per cubic meter of air.

MOLD

Think dry. Buy a dehumidifier for your bedroom and any other room you spend a lot of time in during warm and wet months. Molds need dampness to get busy, so run the bathroom and kitchen fans to fight humidity. (Dust mites also thrive in humidity but don't fare well when humidity is below 50 percent.)

Give a kid a job. Hire a neighborhood teen to rake your leaves in fall, which will cut down on your exposure to mold spores.

PET DANDER

Bathe your pet. We wouldn't think of telling you to show poor Whiskers the door or to put up one of those sorry-looking adoption posters and wave a tearful farewell to your pet—excuse us, *animal companion*. Instead, all you really need is to keep its dander down. There are special rinses and moisturizing cleaners that can help. Allerpet/D (for dogs) and Allerpet/C (for cats) are de-allergenic moisturizers that reduce your pet's flaky behavior. They are available through your veterinarian.

Wait a minute. Bathe your cat? It can be done, insists Marvin Samuelson, D.V.M., director of the Animal Dermatology and Allergy Clinic in Topeka, Kansas. "Cats are apprehensive about water, but after a few times, they get used to it," he says. "Just don't try to fight with the cat. It'll win."

Pick the right pet. If you don't own a pet but want one, be aware that some varieties give out less dander than others. In general, dogs with thick, heavy coats such as English sheepdogs and Pomeranians will hold more dust and dander in their fur, making them more allergy evoking. (The same goes for cats.) On the other hand, says Dr. Samuelson, the short-haired Chihuahua has been held up as the closest thing to a hypoallergenic dog. Those looking for something a little more on the macho side might consider a nice boa constrictor.

IN GENERAL

Limit your bad habits. Smoking and drinking can worsen allergies. Alcohol, because it dilates the blood ves-

• •

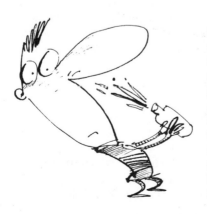

Hot and Clear

Capsaicin, the chemical that adds the fire to hot peppers, may help clear chronically stuffed-up noses, says allergist Alkis Toglas, M.D., of Johns Hopkins Asthma and Allergy Research Center. He is testing the ingredient in nasal inhalants, with encouraging results. A few fiery blasts, and your nose runs like Niagara.

sels, can increase the severity of your runny nose and watery eyes. And because it's a depressant, it mixes especially poorly with sedating over-the-counter antihistamines. Smoking, of course, will further irritate your eyes and respiratory tract and can bring on an asthma attack.

Claim sanctuary. You can't steer clear of all allergens all the time. But even so, it pays to designate one room in your house (most likely the bedroom or anywhere you spend most of your free time) as an allergy-free zone. Air-condition the room, keep it free of carpeting and upholstery, and lock out the cat. By choosing one room and ridding it of allergens, you may be able to improve your condition. "Constant exposure to an allergen can make the nose a chronically irritated organ," says Thomas Platts-Mills, M.D., head of the Division of Allergy and Immunology at the University of Virginia Medical Center in Charlottesville. For example, you might have a minor allergy to your pet that doesn't bother you most of the year, but when your nose is chronically irritated in hay fever season, even a brief encounter with a cat or dog can trigger a sneezing fit.

MEDICATIONS

If none of the above is providing adequate relief, there are a number of over-the-counter remedies for hay fever that can help you through occasional allergy attacks. These come in two general categories: antihistamines and decongestants.

Antihistamines work by stopping histamine from reaching receptor cells in the mucous membranes, thereby blocking the symptoms of hay fever. Over-the-counter antihistamines such as Benadryl and Chlor-Trimeton have a sedating effect, so if you're taking a long drive, pop open a box of tissues instead.

Decongestants, often included in antihistamine medications, constrict blood vessels and cause the mucous membranes to shrink. Decongestants have a stimulant effect, which may counteract the sedation of an antihistamine but also may simply make you nervous as well as tired. Other potential drawbacks include accelerated heartbeat, insomnia and an aggravation of any existing prostate trouble.

Once you start taking a medication, stick with it. A common mistake, says Dr. Storms, is that people take an antihistamine, feel better and ignore the instructions on the label. Just because you feel fine doesn't mean you should discontinue use.

If your old medicine doesn't seem to be doing the trick anymore, try switching brands. "It's not been proven," Dr. Platts-Mills says, "but many patients say that they seem to build up an immunity to their antihistamines."

Dr. Storms advises that you read the labels of any medications for active ingredients. Most brands use chlorpheniramine, which is fine for most people, but if it's not effective for you, try switching to a different active ingredient, such as clemastine (an antihistamine newly available over the

• •

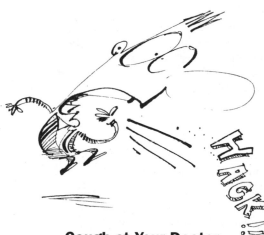

Cough at Your Doctor

Coughs from colds usually fade away after one or two weeks in otherwise healthy people. But if your hack is getting worse or hanging on, see a physician. "A persistent cough without explanation may signal something else," says Emil Bardana, M.D., of the Oregon Health Sciences University School of Medicine. Like what else? Anything from bronchitis and asthma to, in rarer cases, tuberculosis, lung cancer and heart disease. Or perhaps the cough is being triggered by an airborne irritant at work or at home. "Each case must be treated individually," stresses Dr. Bardana. Your doctor will examine you and consider your medical history and occupation; then he may order a chest x-ray. Meanwhile, don't be alarmed by a cough. It's your body's natural reflex for keeping your airways clear. Just see a doctor if it won't go away.

counter and used in the brand Tavist-D).

If you're not getting relief from the drugstore shelves, or if the drowsiness that can accompany medication is bringing you down, ask your doctor to prescribe a nonsedating antihistamine such as Seldane or Hismanal. Be sure to follow the recommended dosage and to inform your doctor if you are on antibiotics—some antibiotics can boost the amount of antihistamine in the blood, causing potentially dangerous heart arrhythmia. In an effort to combat this, researchers at Georgetown University are testing a Seldane metabolite (the compound that the liver metabolizes Seldane into), which appears to block histamine with no adverse side effects.

Those who want to avoid popping pills can ask for a prescription steroid nasal spray, such as Vancenase or Nasacort, which, like other steroids, helps reduce inflammation. But this is strictly a topical application, says Dr. Storms—it does not have the many side effects such as increased blood pressure, bone loss and organ damage that the steroid pushers down at the gym are at risk for. Corticosteroid treatment should be started a few days before the onset of an allergy season. Some patients do complain of nosebleeds or a stinging sensation.

Cromolyn sodium, another prescription spray, is used to stabilize the cells that normally release histamine, effectively shutting down the problem at its site. The drug has no side effects, says Dr. Storms, but it must be used as many as five times a day to prevent the onset of allergy symptoms.

SHOTS

Your doctor may also recommend immunotherapy, or allergy shots. Small amounts of the substance you're allergic to are injected, in ever-increasing doses, once or twice a week until a "maintenance level" is reached—the highest dose tolerable without causing a severe reaction. Once that level has been reached (which takes about two to four months), boosters can be given every one to three weeks. After four to six years at the maintenance level, shots are generally discontinued. About 80 percent of people who undergo immunotherapy remain relatively allergy-free for life, although some therapy patients find themselves slowly sliding back into the sniffling mode.

While the exact mechanism behind allergy shots is not fully understood, it is believed that exposing the body to low levels of the antigen trains the immune system to not respond to higher levels and to not release histamine.

No matter what triggers them, allergies are a hassle. But that doesn't mean you should curse your immune system every time you have a bout of sneezing. "Allergies aren't a weakness; they're a strength," says Bob Lanier, M.D., an allergist in Fort Worth, Texas. "When someone says 'I have allergies,' what they're really saying is 'I have a superior immune system.' " He points out that allergies served to protect early man from parasites and that, anecdotally at least, people with allergies do seem to have fewer health problems in other areas.

And that's nothing to sneeze at.

Cutting-Edge Surgery

Pinholes instead of incisions. Band-Aids instead of scars. Welcome to the brave new world of scalpel-free operations.

•••••••••••••••••••

TIME WAS, FIXING A HERNIA would have meant serious trouble for a guy like Eddie Brown, wide receiver for the Cincinnati Bengals. Sure, it's a routine operation, often done with just a local anesthetic. Nevertheless, it usually requires a five-inch cut across the lower abdomen and six weeks off work to recover. When Brown's hernia was diagnosed, he expected to be sidelined the rest of the season. "I really wanted to get back," Brown says. "I love to play."

To help him do it, the Bengals' team physician sent Brown to Boyd Crafton, an M.D. at the University of Cincinnati who could do the operation a new way. Instead of making a big incision to reach Brown's abdominal rupture,

Dr. Crafton made three small holes. In one hole, he stuck a flexible tube called a laparoscope, which has a tiny camera on the end of it, so he could look inside Brown's body. In the other holes, he inserted special tools that are manipulated from outside the body to attach a piece of rupture-patching mesh over the hernia. Afterward, the punctures were covered with those little adhesive dot bandages. Less than two weeks later, Brown played against the New York Giants in one of his best games of the season.

Stories like Eddie Brown's are becoming more and more common for men from all walks of life. Using an expanding array of tubes, scopes, catheters and miniature tools, surgeons are now able to avoid incisions when diagnosing or fixing some of the most common problems men suffer from. Among these are prostate cancer, clogged arteries, gallstone attacks and overuse injuries to joints. So many of these procedures are being developed that experts are calling it a revolution that may someday make the scalpel obsolete.

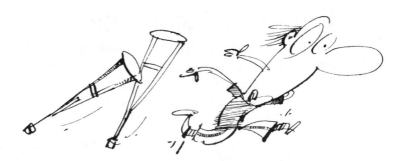

Fun with Your New Knees

It used to be thought that following reconstructive knee surgery, you had to rest for 6 to 12 weeks before doing any vigorous exercise. But a new program developed at the Center for Athletic Medicine in Chicago allows knee surgery patients to start running after only 6 weeks. Aggressive exercise speeds the healing process, according to the center's director, Preston Wolin, M.D.: "We start exercising the patient as soon as he wakes up—the body likes it."

FASTER RECOVERY

The main advantage of no-scalpel techniques is that they can put you back on your feet up to five times faster than traditional surgeries. "In any operation, it's the incision that really slows you down afterward," says Lee Swanstrom, M.D., director of minimally invasive surgery at Holladay Park Medical Center in Portland, Oregon. "If you avoid the incision, you avoid its drawbacks—pain, time in the hospital and time off work."

While many of these less-invasive procedures take longer to perform than a traditional operation done with a scalpel, the cost is often much lower because recovery is quicker. Used diagnostically, no-scalpel methods sometimes eliminate the need for surgery altogether.

Most of the new techniques involve *endoscopy,* which refers to any procedure that allows a doctor to peer at your innards through a tube. An endoscope is about as big in diameter as a pencil. Endoscopes have different names, depending on where they're used in the body. When used in joints, for example, they're called arthroscopes; when used in the abdomen, they're called laparoscopes. By some estimates, 80 percent of all surgeries will be done with one kind of scope or another by the end of the decade.

Scopes aren't really a new idea. Even at the turn of the century, doctors were peering through the body's natural openings with crude rigid tubes to see, for example, the bladder, colon and stomach. When fiber optics came along, tiny lenses and magnifiers could be placed on the tips of scopes, providing much clearer views. Miniature video cameras now let doctors see things bigger than life on a monitor. (During surgery, this creates the disconcerting impression that everybody in the operating room is ignoring the patient to watch TV.) The precision of fiber optics also makes it feasible to use lasers to cut and seal tissue. And just as optics improved, surgeons' tools became smaller and more flexible, allowing easier access to more places in the body.

FIX UP THIS JOINT

Joints are a case in point. Arthroscopy got its start in the knees, which are like little caverns filled with fluid. Surgeons have plenty of space to work under the kneecap and can easily use tools to repair torn cartilage and ligaments, remove bone chips or smooth out rough spots. Arthroscopic knee surgery has been a godsend to thousands of active men who've demanded too much of their knees. Now they can have surgery on Saturday, spend Sunday on crutches and be back at work on Monday. In some cases, they can return to running or tennis about a month into a physical therapy program. It was once normal to spend three weeks on crutches after an "open" knee procedure, according to James Fox, M.D., a surgeon at Southern California Orthopedic Institute. "The only disadvantage in the new method is that despite having had major surgery, you get no sympathy from your friends, since you're taking no medications and have no scars," says Dr. Fox.

Now, as arthroscopy equipment becomes smaller still, doctors are able to make repairs in tighter joints such as shoulders, ankles, elbows, hips and toes. In the jaw, surgeons use scopes to diagnose and treat painful disorders of the temporomandibular joint, which is about one-tenth the size of the knee.

Having space in which to work is important in all scope procedures. In the abdomen, for example, where organs press tightly together, a new procedure has doctors inflate the belly with carbon dioxide gas to create a tentlike space. Peer inside, and the organs are laid out like a page from an anatomy textbook.

NO SCARS

This advance makes it possible to do laparoscopic procedures such as gallbladder removal, which 147,000 men undergo each year. If Lyndon B. Johnson could have had his gallbladder surgery today, he wouldn't have had that impressive scar across his belly to show off for White House photographers. In fact, gallbladder operations are what really got the no-scalpel revolution going, surgeons say. A scant four years after the first laparoscopic one was done, about 75 percent of all gallbladder removals are performed without incisions. Patient enthusiasm led doctors to become proficient with scopes, paving the way for advances in operations that men undergo even more, such as hernia repair. Today, no-scalpel techniques are also used to:

Treat prostate problems. Each year, an estimated 400,000 prostates are removed, usually when the gland becomes cancerous. "If cancer has already spread beyond the prostate, there's no point in taking it out or treating it with radiation," says Louis Kavoussi, M.D., assistant professor of urology at Harvard Medical School. To decide on the right treatment, urologists using a laparoscope can sample nearby lymph glands to tell if the cancer has spread.

Operations to trim an enlarged prostate can now be done with lasers, which may cause less bleeding and allow quicker recovery. The devices are being evaluated by the Food and Drug Administration but are already available and in use at many major hospitals.

Unclog arteries. As an alternative to bypass surgery, doctors make a small incision, usually in the groin, and thread a specially outfitted catheter to the site of the blockage. One kind of tool destroys obstructing plaque with pulses of laser light. Another uses a spinning V-shaped blade to drill through deposits and pump out the residue. Still another device props open cleared-out blood vessels by implanting a tiny stainless steel mesh that expands inside the artery.

Repair the back. Tissue that's leaked out of a ruptured disk can be trimmed and removed with special cutting and vacuuming tools, relieving the pressure on adjacent nerves in the spine. It's done with only a local anesthetic, and patients are active again in a week, according to the Texas Back Institute.

Remove cancer. Surgeons have begun to take tumors from the lungs, neck, bowel and kidneys endoscopically. However, some doctors fear that cancer may spread when tumors are pulled through the body to the surgical hole. These operations may become more common as follow-up studies are completed over the next several years.

Perform vasectomies. No scopes involved here—the semen-bearing vas lies right next to the surface of the scrotum. Still, extracting the vas for cutting and tying through a small puncture instead of a cut is more comfortable for patients, takes fewer steps, can be done in 15 minutes instead of the customary 45 and requires no stitches. "The experience is no more unpleasant than giving blood," says urologist Maurice Sandler, M.D., chief of surgery at Brookside Hospital in San Pablo, California.

Heal ulcers. Endoscopes are used primarily to diagnose ulcers and occasionally to stop ulcers from bleeding. Lasers can be used in conjunction with endoscopes to stop bleeding, although this application is relatively new.

Relieve sinuses. By using a tiny scope to clear sinuses blocked by bone spurs, polyps or swelling, doctors significantly reduce damage to the sinus lining and keep pain and bleeding at a minimum.

No-scalpel procedures aren't always the best choice. Some critics charge that scopes are being put into use so fast that nobody can be sure they really work better in the long run. Plus, doctors admit endoscopy takes some getting used to, which puts a premium on training and experience. "It's like playing an advanced version of Nintendo," says Howard Winfield, M.D., a University of Iowa urologist who teaches other doctors. "Some surgeons may not have the patient load necessary to maintain the skills."

The consensus is that patients should choose for themselves. "All I would ask a critic is how he wants his own operation done," says urologist Ralph Clayman, M.D. "Knowing what I know, if I needed to have a kidney removed for benign disease, it would be done laparoscopically." If you're a candidate for a no-scalpel operation, experts suggest you:

■ Ask your doctor how much experience he has with the procedure. In general, he should have at least 25 similar operations under his belt—fewer if the technique is new and not frequently used. (Ten ulcer operations, for instance, is a lot.)

■ Inquire about long-term results. What's known about complications? Is there a chance of needing another operation to do the job over?

You can also ask the opinion of a patient who's already gone under the no-knife. Take Eddie Brown, for example. Of his return to the playing field to run 107 yards when he otherwise would have been bedridden, he says simply, "I felt *good*."

—*Richard Laliberte*

Part 7

LOOKING GOOD

Grooming 101

Want to make your appearance a class act?
Use this shampoo-to-shoes grooming guide for men.

••••••••••••••••••••

AN OLD HIGH-SCHOOL BUDDY came for a stay a while ago. Tough guy. Kind of guy who knows what's important in life. Beer. Sports. John Deere caps. Then he walked into my bathroom and caught me in a compromising position with a can of hair spray and my wife's bristle brush. If I had simply been, oh, wearing a tutu and crooning "I Feel Pretty," our friendship might have survived intact, but the look of disgust on his face told me things would never be the same. Yet at the risk of being labeled a dandy, I freely admit that I am conscious about my appearance. And good grooming is a significant part of that, critical for small but important matters such as flirting with waitresses, courting business associates or asking for long-overdue salary increases.

My general grooming ritual begins with the basics.

Shower. As far as I'm concerned, the only reason there's a bathtub in our apartment is so that my wife has a place to go when football season starts. Showering every day is fine, as long as you don't run the hot water at the upper echelons of your pain endurance. Moderately hot water will clean just as well, according to Allison Vidimos, M.D., staff dermatologist at the Cleveland Clinic Foundation in Cleveland, and if you're creating a steam room every time you shower, you're also drying your skin. You can use any type of soap or shower gel you like, but be aware that antibacterial (deodorant) soaps can dry the skin.

Moisturizer. Rubbing on moisturizer may seem about even with synchronized swimming on the testosterone scale, but being from the Northeast, I find I need to use a moisturizer in winter to keep my shoulders from becoming dry and making the act of putting on a shirt a rather painful ordeal. Towel-dry lightly, then apply a simple, scent-free moisturizing lotion. "Stay away from anything that claims to revitalize, stop aging or contain collagen, placental extract or amniotic fluid," warns Dr. Vidimos. I can usually convince my wife to rub a lotion on my back and shoulders, but if you're on your own, try wrapping plain cotton gauze around the end of a ruler or back scratcher and using the gauze as an applicator to reach the middle of your back.

Deodorant. I find that right after the shower is the best time to put on a deodorant, since, having the attention span of a three-year-old, I am often adjusting the knot in my tie before realizing I've forgotten this basic step. Trying to negotiate a stick of deodorant between the buttons of your dress shirt and up under your jacketed arm takes more dexterity than most of us have at 7:30 in the morning. When it comes to choosing what to wear under your arms, roll-on, stick or spray concoctions are all a matter of choice. What's most important is whether you use a deodorant, an antiperspirant or a combination of both. An antiperspirant will keep you from sweating but do nothing for your odor; a deodorant will smite your BO but not your sweat. To be dry *and* odor-free, be sure your choice is labeled "deodorant/antiperspirant." And remember to dry your underarms thoroughly before you apply it. It's designed to keep you dry, not make you that way.

Colognes. Once you've taken away your own scent, you may want to add someone else's, be it Calvin's, Ralph's or Giorgio's. Less is more—if you leave a puddle when you stand still, perhaps you're laying it on a bit heavy. Fortunately, most men's fragrance manufacturers have been kind enough to discourage us from overindulgence by making their products incredibly expensive. Cologne is alcohol-based, so keep it away from sensitive skin, such as the armpit, groin or freshly shaved face, warns Jerome Shupack, M.D., professor of clinical dermatology at the New York University School of Medicine. I generally put the smallest of drops behind my ears, at the base of my throat and at my wrists. Apply your cologne a good 10 or 15 minutes before you leave the house, so it will have time to dry and won't be quite so pungent when the carpool pulls up.

SHAVING POINTS

For clean shaving, a sharp razor is a must. Trying to save money by using a disposable razor or blade more than three or four times is not a good investment, because all your savings will go toward tissue paper for blotting the bleeding nicks you've left on your face. If the razor pulls at your beard when you run it against your face, it needs to be replaced.

Preparation. Shower before you shave, as the steam will soften your beard and make the whole process easier. Moisturizing the beard is the most important thing a shaving medium can do, and most shaving creams will do the trick quite well. I've tried soap, which works to a fair degree, but a moisturizer will do in a pinch if you apply it to a wet face. One friend of mine even admitted that in an emergency, he was forced to use olive oil and found it actually quite effective.

The stroke. Stroke gently, drawing the razor slowly in the direction your beard grows. Shave smooth areas first and save the difficult parts of your face, such as under the chin, for last. That gives the shaving cream more time to take effect. Pay close attention to keeping your sideburns even: Right-handed men tend to shave their left sideburn shorter than their right, and vice versa for southpaws.

Shaving bumps. Many men develop rashes or other problems from shaving. Acnelike pimples in the beard area can be caused by bacteria invading the hair follicles as well as the tiny breaks in the skin caused by shaving, says Dr. Vidimos. These breakouts can be minimized by using a medicated shaving cream, available in drugstores, or by washing the face first with a medicated soap.

Ingrown hairs are a separate problem, especially for African-Americans and for men with very heavy beards. "They're caused by the razor shaving the hair shaft into a point," Dr. Shupack says. If you're having a problem with ingrown hairs, be especially careful not to shave against the grain, and do always use a sharp blade. Switching to an electric razor may help, but many men find the only way to solve the problem is to join the ranks of the bearded.

After-shaves. Traditional after-shaves are alcohol-based, so splashing them on after shaving usually causes a stinging sensation that earlier, more pain-tolerant generations of men apparently enjoyed. Personally, if I want my face to sting, I'll make a pass at my wife's sister, but after-shave I can do without. Simple cold water or a moisturizer (one labeled "for facial use") will help soothe your razored skin, and Dr. Shupack has an even better idea: Use a sunscreen on your face right after shaving. Consider: Men are twice as likely as women to get some form of skin cancer. Most sunscreens have a moisturizing ingredient that will soften your skin as well as protect against sun damage. Avoid waterproof sunscreens, which may be greasy.

FACING UP TO PROBLEM SKIN

As an average, pimply-faced kid, I couldn't wait for adulthood to dawn and banish the pox of acne from my visage. My college diploma meant more to me than a shot at a career. It meant I had escaped adolescence and could look forward to a future as a clear-complected grown-up.

I was wrong.

Well, my complexion is somewhat clearer than, say, Jimmy Swaggart's conscience, but I still have to battle with the occasional breakout—blackheads, whiteheads, angry red pimples, a veritable Rainbow Coalition of zits. While these various types of breakouts look dissimilar, they have the same causes and the same cures.

Adult acne can come in two forms, according to Dr. Vidimos. *Acne vulgaris* is a continuation of the teenage affliction. *Acne rosacea,* on the other hand, is an adult-onset acne that usually affects the center of the face, especially the nose and cheeks, and consists of red, inflamed pimples. Dr. Vidimos points to W. C. Fields's swollen red nose as an example. (And I always thought it was the bourbon.)

The causes. The various types of pimples are all a result of dead skin cells plugging the openings to the oil glands of the face, back and chest.

When the top of the plug is exposed to the surface, the air darkens the dead cells, causing a blackhead. When the plug remains below the surface, oil and debris will continue to accumulate in the blocked pore, and as they are broken down by bacteria, an inflammation will occur, eventually

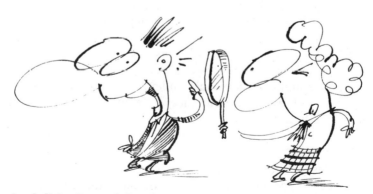

Invisible Sound System

The biggest beef about hearing aids is that they're too bulky and noticeable. But now under study at the California Ear Institute is a tiny hearing aid, smaller than a contact lens. The transmitter attaches to the eardrum with a drop of mineral oil.

blooming into a full-fledged prom buster.

One thing you can do to fight breakouts is take a vacation. Stress has been implicated in eruptions of this nature—though for the record, foods with a reputation for causing pimples, such as chocolate, potato chips and cola, have not. Of course, given the state of the economy, using zits as an excuse to take a few days off might not be the best career move at this time, but there are other measures you can take to fight the breakouts.

The cures. Wash your face with soap and water two or three times a day—say, morning, when you return from work and before bedtime. Use a mild soap to prevent overdrying of the skin. Soaps manufactured especially for problem acne are also available. (You can tell the druggist you're buying it for your daughter.) After each washing, you can further clean your face with those medicated pads sold in drugstores. Be careful, though, as overuse can irritate the skin or cause excess dryness. If you notice dry skin, stop using the pads. Finally, apply a topical cream containing benzoyl peroxide. If, despite your best efforts, acne continues to be a problem, consult a dermatologist for a topical or an oral prescription medication.

Handling a breakout. Dermatologists will tell you that if you get a pimple, you should let it run its course. You, naturally, will ignore this advice—who can tolerate the outrage of a zit in all its glory? Dr. Shupack admits that yes, you can gently try to squeeze a pimple once it's come to a head, but "the problem is that most people don't know when to stop. It becomes almost a personal vendetta." If you can't get the bugger with gentle pressure, leave it alone, or risk potential scarring from your encounter.

HAIR AND NOW

Resigned to the fact that my hair is beginning to go the way of the spotted owl's habitat, I've found that making the most of what I have is a large part of looking my best. Keeping a contemporary hairstyle is an important aspect of that—and maybe the trickiest part of the whole vanity package. I lopped off my ponytail back in 1988, when I realized that I didn't really want Steven Seagal as my fashion role model. The big dilemma today is whether to grow those "90210" sideburns. I'm still hedging.

The haircut. Staying contemporary doesn't mean running to your barber with tear sheets from the fashion magazines. "It's not helpful to say 'Comb it over this way or that way,'" explains Gene Kottas, manager of the barber division at the College of Hair Design in Lincoln, Nebraska. "Some hair will do it, and some won't." If you're unhappy with your current haircut, ask for suggestions. If you're still unhappy, look for a new barber.

Shampooing. Even the sharpest coif needs daily maintenance. If you have oily hair, you'll need to shampoo every day—hair with too much moisture will have an oily sheen to it and will tend to mat against the scalp. Men with dry hair will need to shampoo less—say, every other day. Frizzy hair and an itchy scalp are signs of dryness. Any good-quality shampoo will suffice, but avoid those that claim to condition while they clean. "I don't see how you can condition hair by putting something in and clean it by taking something out at the same time," says Kottas.

Conditioning. Conditioners can do two things: They can add moisture, or they can add protein. Dry hair will appear frizzy and have a strawlike feel to it, but a moisturizing conditioner can help make dry hair as bouncy as a check from your congressman. If your hair tends to break or split at the ends, a protein-enriching conditioner will coat the hair and give you the illusion of thickness. But use it sparingly: Overuse may clog hair follicles and cause them to become inflamed, according to Dr. Vidimos.

Instruments of style. Once out of the shower, you should never use a bristle brush on wet hair—it will snarl and may cause the hair to break. Kottas recommends a vent brush (a plastic brush with airflow holes) or a comb for wet hair.

If using a blow-dryer is just too far off the macho scale for you, you should note that the *Wall Street Journal* recently reported that eight in ten American men blow-dry their hair. So there's no shame in using one, no matter what my old high-school buddy says. However, blow-dryers can damage the hair if not handled properly, suggests Kottas. The problem is not so much the temperature setting (a higher setting will give you a stronger hold) but rather overdrying already dry hair. Hair damaged by dryness can sprout frizzies and split ends and can easily break. Hold the dryer six to ten inches from the head, and keep moving it so that you don't overheat any one spot.

Hair dressings. Dressings come in three forms: lotions, mousses and gels. Lotions will give you a light hold. If you have thin hair like I do, a lotion is all you'll need to keep it in place. Heavier hair requires a styling mousse— which comes in a foam dispenser like whipped cream—or a gel. Some gels can hold your hair stiff enough to audition for the Sex Pistols reunion tour, but your best bet is to try a couple of different products to find just how much hold you require. Put the product on wet hair if you want a longer, stronger hold. Hair sprays will also give you a strong hold but should be used only on hair that's already dried.

Dandruff. No matter how meticulous you are with your hair, a few flakes of dandruff are going to show up on the shoulders of your navy blue Brooks Brothers blazer. People actually slough their skin every 28 days, losing a total of 1 ½ pounds of skin each year, and the scalp is no exception. Minor flakiness can be taken care of by using a rubber scrub brush on your scalp when you shampoo. Severe problems are a different matter.

Seborrheic dermatitis is the clinical term for chronic dandruff, a condition that can affect not just the scalp but also the eyebrows and beard area and can leave a guy looking flakier than a Greenwich Village Halloween. Most likely caused by an inflammation of the oil glands in the face and scalp, severe dandruff can be aggravated by stress, allergy attacks or illness and tends to be worse in winter than summer.

There are several over-the-counter dandruff shampoos with zinc, tar, salicylic acid or selenium and sulfur as active ingredients, all which work more or less as well as the others. Try one or two of these remedies first, and if the problem doesn't abate, consult your doctor for a topical steroid lotion to fight the inflammation. Soaps containing sulfur or zinc are also available for use on the face.

Facial hair. Deciding to grow a beard or mustache is a momentous decision (although not as momentous as shav-

ing one off). A beard can minimize the effect of facial fea-
tures such as a large nose or weak chin. After about a month
of growth, you'll want to start shaping the new beard,
according to *Lia Schorr's Skin Care Guide for Men*. First,
shave your neck, making a clean line under your chin; then
shave your cheeks. You'll need to shave the edges daily
unless you want to start looking like a Mennonite. Also, you
need to shampoo the beard daily, a process easily accom-
plished in the shower. Once a week, trim it using special
beard-cutting scissors, available in a cutlery store. Brush the
beard up, then down, to get out tangles before cutting. Also,
always trim your beard when it's dry. Cut a wet beard, and
it's sure to dry out lopsided.

WATCH YOUR MOUTH

As everyone knows, the most difficult part about dental
care is inventing original and yet vaguely believable excuses
for putting off your next visit to the dentist. There are easy
ways out, such as "There's a big seminar on tape dispensers
I just have to catch" or "Damn, that's the day Geraldo is
doing 'When Hermaphrodites Kill.' "

Regardless of your creativity, you're going to have to
visit your dentist sometime—twice a year in most cases,

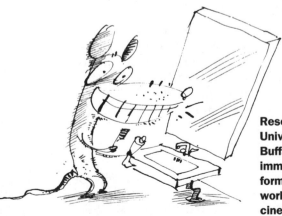

Gum Shots

**Researchers at the State
University of New York at
Buffalo have succeeded in
immunizing rats against a
form of periodontal disease,
work that could lead to a vac-
cine to immunize humans
against the leading cause of
adult tooth loss.**

more often if you're having any problems with your teeth or gums. But the way in which you care for your own teeth is the most important aspect of keeping a healthy mouth, clean breath and a winning smile.

The basics they taught us in junior-high health class still apply: Brushing and flossing after each meal cleans your teeth of plaque, that thin, colorless, sticky film that forms on your masticators and holds food particles to them. When you eat sugars or starches, the bacteria in the plaque interact with the food particles to produce acids, which break down tooth enamel and form cavities in the teeth. Neglect the plaque, and next thing you know, you're feet-up in a dentist's chair with a jackhammer probing your gum line.

Brushing. In a word: gentle. A soft-bristled brush will clean your teeth better than a hard one will, because the bristles give against the tooth enamel, expanding to surround the entire tooth. Soft bristles will also be much gentler on your gums.

Toothpastes. The truly trendy have already switched to baking soda toothpaste, which leaves the mouth tasting somewhat salty. Sarah Turner, president of the American Dental Hygienists Association and an instructor at the Hawkeye Institute of Technology in Waterloo, Iowa, says that baking soda neutralizes acids from plaque and may have some positive effect on gingivitis. Turner also says that tartar control toothpastes seem to work. Just be sure that any paste you use also contains fluoride—a proven cavity fighter.

Breath control. Mouthwashes work okay, and so does chewing on a stick of sugarless gum. But here's a trick an old coworker taught me for business meals. Order a salad with whole radishes, and set the radishes aside until you're done. Noshing on them will freshen your breath just as well.

HELPING HANDS

Even though modern man no longer uses his nails for clawing through dirt and tearing into enemies (we have divorce lawyers for that), knowing how to care for them properly is still important.

Cleaning. Simply washing your hands often isn't

enough to get dirt out from under your nails. You can buy a flat, hard-bristled nail brush to rub against the edges of your fingernails and clean out any debris. Achieve the same effect and win kudos from your housemate by doing the dishes.

Simple manicure. Some men spend a great deal of time tending their nails, filing them every day and applying clear nail polish. These men usually wear diamond pinky rings and try to sell the rest of us land deals in Florida. But a simple home manicure is a good idea, especially if you have bitten or damaged cuticles (the opaque skin folds at the base of your nails). Soak your hands in warm water for a few minutes first. After the cuticles soften, gently push them back using your fingernail, a washcloth or a cuticle pusher. If the cuticle bunches, trim the excess flesh with a cuticle clipper, which is similar to a small scissors but has blades that meet evenly rather than overlap. Properly trimmed cuticles will show off the lunule, that whitish half-moon of living tissue at the base of the nail.

Trimming. Trim both toenails and fingernails straight across to prevent ingrown nails. If the edges of the nails are rough, use an emery board or nail file to file them down. File from the outside toward the center, Dr. Vidimos says. And be certain to ever so slightly round off the corners of your toenails with a file or nail scissors, lest your bedmate begin complaining of pierced ankles.

Grooming is as important as a firm handshake when it comes to making a good impression, and the basics of grooming are simple rules anyone can follow. In fact, I happened to see my friend from high school recently. I noticed he had not only a new haircut but a meticulously trimmed goatee. I asked him out for a beer, but he said he had to get home.

Needed his beauty rest, he said.

—Stephen Perrine

Blue Blazer of Glory

*An ode to the navy blazer,
the one indispensable part of a man's wardrobe.*

• • • • • • • • • • • • • • • • • •

THE GHOST OF CHRISTMAS FUTURE, disguised cleverly as the neighbor boy, stopped by the other day.

Since I live in a small house surrounded by rampant vegetation and declining agriculture, neighbors are a novelty. I used to live in New York City. If your neighbor stopped by, you called the police. Around here, you yell "Come in!" and figure it out later.

"I need some advice," the neighbor boy said from downstairs.

There was a bat in the attic at the time. Bats cheese me off. I know they have admirers: Author Tom Robbins used to answer his telephone with an unrequested discourse on bat mystique. Mike Nichols, the adventurer-photographer, belongs to some bat fan club. I saw both Batman movies. I just don't get it. To me, bats seem as if they were made to provide air cover for rats, and I feel a compelling need to defeat them, vanquish them utterly as part of my bit for all mankind.

But even more than I feel a need to kill bats, I feel a compulsion to pontificate, to dispense far more advice than required. I can't resist it. My second-favorite sentences all start with the phrase "What do you think . . . " My favorite sentences all start with the phrase "What you ought to do is . . . " Advice is me.

Add to that the almost overwhelming desire felt by men of a certain age to pass on avuncular wisdom to teenage boys, and you have all you need to make your own backyard windbag. There's an obvious reason for this, by the way. It's because all of us suffered our most painful slings and arrows while still in the clutches of puberty. For example, adolescence is when you freeze your taste in women, choosing as your model of ideal beauty, in the manner of a lovestruck Browning, the girl *just out of reach*. You discover the red line on your humiliation meter in high school and make your first big mistakes. Something inside all us post-teen chumps wants to rewrite that part of the script, to undo the bad stuff and make it possible to score at last with the cheerleader of our dreams.

So on those rare occasions when a teenage kid says he'll actually listen to my oracular pronouncements, I'm out of the attic pronto. I forgot the bat, and I went down the stairs and into the kitchen where the neighbor boy was standing, leaning on the open door of my refrigerator.

"What's up?"

"I've got to get my picture taken for school," he said, dragging a slice of pizza from the middle shelf, peeling off the congealed pepperoni slices and popping them into his mouth as if they were the dinner mints of Attila.

"And?"

"They say I need a dark coat." Yow, the whole slice in two bites. I waited. "What do you think I ought to buy?"

PICTURE PERFECT

The neighbor boy is 16 and is gaining in horizontality what I already possess in verticality. So we could share a size, more or less. At least we're close enough for high-school portraiture. "What you ought to do is get a blazer," I pronounced. "Until you do, I've got just what you need." I ran back up and produced a navy blue blazer made by a venerable manufacturer back in the days when people remembered the *Pueblo.*

He tried it on, a perfect fit, an instant transformation.

"Buy one of these."

He was nervous. He slipped in front of a mirror and looked at himself sideways. It embarrassed him, and he quickly took it off. "How come a suit coat?"

"No, no, *no,* my young turnip. This is a *jacket,* a blazer to be precise, and not a coat"—an easy distinction, but one not found in dictionaries—"and it's exactly the thing." I piled on a white shirt and a necktie decorated in neutral blandness, patted him on the back and showed him the door. "Bathe first."

Neighbor boy goes away, comes back a few days later

dressed in jeans, open high-tops, Metallica T-shirt. In a grocery sack, he's got my blazer, tie and shirt. In his other hand, he's got pictures. On my front porch, neighbor boy looks like a methadone-and-motorcycle man. But in the pictures, he looks like the young executive down at the bank who keeps turning down my loan requests.

"I need a jacket like this," he says. Then he adds, in an almost inaudible, semireflective, pubescent whisper, "It's sort of grown-up."

It was one of those mileposts, like the day you decide you really don't mind cauliflower. He actually liked wearing the blazer. It was like shaking hands with the twisted sister of respectability backstage after the concert. It made him feel good because it made him feel important—made him feel like a man. Nothing permanent, mind you. Just a mild flirtation with grown-uphood. But enough to make him realize he needed something like a navy blazer as a kind of fallback, in case being a teenager wasn't the career we all thought it was.

• •

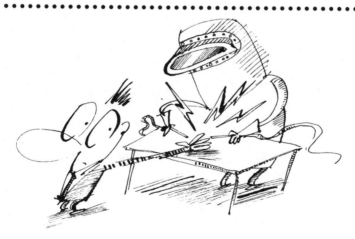

Wart Zapper

Nobody likes warts, and now there's a new way to get rid of them called controlled localized heating. Doctors have found that passing a mild electrical current through a wart can make it shrink. A study of the technique found it to be an effective de-warter more than 80 percent of the time.

SUITS DON'T SUIT ME

"It's like a suit," he said. Like a suit, but with none of the downside of suitdom. Suits spell well-dressed incompetence to a young man of cynical disposition. Suits mean you're a thief and a scoundrel but you still want approval. For example, all congressmen wear suits. *Real thugs* don't care. You don't need a suit to rob a 7-Eleven. You need a suit to rob the U.S. Treasury.

So I'm giving him the blazer for Christmas, because he's right. He needs a jacket like that. A navy blue blazer is the one indispensable part of a man's wardrobe. And while the neighbor boy doesn't realize it, he's standing next to the abyss, a 16-year old right on the perilous brink of manhood, where armies meet in boardrooms and on shop floors by day and where all the officers wear blazers by night. My first blazer was also a Christmas gift, and I remember putting it on and seeing past the edge of childhood all the way to a first mortgage. Gave me the willies, I don't mind saying.

The military aspect of a blazer isn't incidental, incidentally. From its ancestor, the outer doublet of the fifteenth century—from which we have also derived windbreakers, trench coats and tuxedo and varsity jackets—the blazer detoured through a hitch in the navy followed by a long tenure at English boarding schools, where the upper classes were given a genteel paramilitary costume to wear before they were shipped off to the trenches of the Crimea. Things are tamer now, of course. These days blazers are corporate fatigues. If the Episcopal Church had an army, buck-private vergers would all be wearing navy blazers.

Maybe its quasimilitary history is what contributes to the blazer's inherent nattiness. Neighbor boy—soon to be *Mr.* Boy—liked my blazer because he could go grown-up in increments. This year, he might dress up a pair of jeans and some high-tops simply by putting on a pale blue shirt, a tie and a blazer. He could be a grown-up from the waist up, where maturity and authority count. But he could still be a kid from the waist down, where being young counts even more. Later, the neighbor boy might want to complete the wardrobe by adding a pair of chinos for day and gray wool slacks for night. He'll avoid polyester like the plague it is.

And eventually, he'll want to ditch the high-tops for a pair of dark brown—not *black,* mind you—shoes. Normal shoes. Like the kind Dad wears, unless your dad came of age in the 1960s, in which case you should show him this little article right away.

BLAZER LORE

You didn't ask, but let me give you the same blazer lore I gave the kid next door: Go middle-of-the-road, blazer-wise. For example, I think a double-breasted blazer with six buttons in front and four on each sleeve and double vents in back does nothing but give every man the opportunity to look like the admiral of ice cream. You can get blazers with a streamlined single-button front, and you can get them with a modest two-button sleeve. Twenty-five years ago, chaps were buying Nehru blazers, and when they wore them, they could have passed for drum majors at Kitchener High.

A smart guy buying a blazer will get the government-issue standard model, with two or three buttons in front and a modest number—three to be exact—on each sleeve. Other blazers may have more glory or more flash, but the traditional model has been in style now for 50 years and seems likely to remain in fashion until loincloths make a comeback. A decent blazer shows that you play for the shirts side against the barbarians from the skins team. In the world of perfect men, only guys with well-defined rules about responsibility, duty and tolerance wear blazers. Guys who see life as a long sequence of squeezed weenies don't.

So the kid next door will get his end-of-the-year stripes from me: a navy blazer, the mess dress of the modern man, where fair play, drinks at 6:00 in the evening, woman trouble, golf and insurance binders all mix in life's big soup. I say cheers to him, that well-dressed kid in high-tops. Because starting next year, he'll not only have a decent blazer, he'll also leave school, start figuring out college and girlfriends and generally increase the scope for potential requests for advice, all which bodes well for me. But bodes better for the bats.

—Denis Boyles

Fashion Primer

A man's style is either the smartest or the dumbest thing he can say about himself. Here's how to tell the difference.

● ● ● ● ● ● ● ● ● ● ● ● ● ● ● ● ● ● ●

WHETHER SOMEONE ELSE IS doing the buying or they're doing it themselves, smart men have the solution to the fashion dilemma: Forget fashion. Wear clothes. For the distinction between the two is what marks the difference between a regular guy and an insecure yahoo. Fashion tries very hard to make a statement. Clothes make the man.

Once a man steps out of his clothes and into fashion, he's only a trend-step away from ridicule and social oblivion, his own identity slipping out of his hands and into the paws of trend-mavens. In the final analysis, when we wear clothes, we should also want to wear a little common sense.

How to avoid self-parody in your own life? Here are some notes to take with you when you go shopping—or to pass on to whoever goes for you.

Style. A man's style is either the smartest or the dumbest thing he can say about himself. It is his declaration of self.

How to tell fashion from clothes. If you bought it, it's clothes. If your wife bought it, it's fashion as seen in *Esquire.* Last year. If your girlfriend bought it, it's fashion as seen in *GQ.* This year. If your girlfriend's a manicurist, it's fashion as seen in *Details.* This week.

Guys who try too hard vs. guys who don't. If you can't tell who's trying to be fashionable and who's just being himself, you obviously don't know what to look for. Take a lesson: First, you'll notice how the guys who try too hard seem to be squirming under the weight of fashion, while the guys who know better just show up, do their job and call it a day. Instead of following Arsenio's lead, consider, for example, David Letterman's. The virtue of guys who don't try too hard is their appeal to our common sense. They seem unpretentious, secure and, best of all, rock-solid reliable.

You can't really blame guys who try too hard, though. They're not just fashionable; they're fashion victims. How to avoid becoming one? To increase efficiency, reduce redundancy and ensure your ability to dress in good taste even while temporarily blinded by a hangover, may we offer . . .

A SENSIBLE WARDROBE FOR THE SENSIBLE MAN

The most basic way to avoid a surplus of the wrong kind of clothing is to make sure you don't have room for it. Fill your closet with the stuff you really need to get through life as a well-dressed person, and nothing else will fit.

What You Need

■ Suits of a nonoffensive variety. Specifically, a plain charcoal gray wool suit, a dark blue pinstripe suit (but keep the stripes subtle), a light summer suit and, if you live in a cold climate, a tweed. Get all three-pieces, if you can. Loose-fitting coat; straight-leg trousers with a maximum of two pleats.

■ Navy blue blazer. Specs: three gold buttons on each cuff, two- or three-button front, center fart flap.

■ Plain white and light blue all-cotton long-sleeved shirts (for business).

■ Work shirts made from heavy-gauge cotton.

■ Trousers. Two pairs of chinos or cords, two pairs of denims, two pairs of wool trousers, two pairs of summer-weight wool trousers.

■ Suspenders that button to your pants. This piece of rigging can make a pair of trousers quite comfortable, particularly if you've got more of a middle than you'd like. Makes pants hang nicely, too. Just don't go getting up a head of steam and calling them "braces," as Larry King does.

■ Footwear. Pair of brown oxfords, pair of black or dark brown loafers, pair of work or hiking boots, one pair of sneaks (jogging, exercise, whatever).

■ Fooling-around clothes, including a pair of cutoffs, since recycling is always in style. Also: basic shorts, a T-shirt or two, a decent set of plain sweats and a pair of all-purpose cross-trainers.

What You Don't Need

■ Suits with a plaid, stripe or print visible from more than six feet away. Long, low coat and deeply pleated slacks with legs more than three feet wide and collapsed over the top of the shoes.

■ Sport coats made from synthetic materials or any jacket in a primary color.

■ Business shirts that were made for dirtier business than driving a desk. So no office use of multicolored golf shirts, flannel shirts, madras or army-surplus shirts.

■ Dress shirts worn as work shirts.

■ Pants in safety colors—neon green, hot pink and so on. Sansabelt? Don't even think about it. And sweatpants should never be seen in an office.

■ Suspenders that clip to your pants. And all those cute Daffy Duck and other animal print suspenders.

■ Shoes that call attention to the feet. Also: Unless you're under 17, slip out of those high-top lace-ups worn unlaced, those shoes with jewelry attached and those plastic shoes.

■ Leisurewear, or whatever they used to call this stuff before leisure broke a sweat. Unless you're a professional athlete with a fab physique, stay miles from anything in Lycra spandex.

SOME NOTES ON A SENSIBLE WARDROBE

Men's clothes are, for the most part, better made than women's, with far greater attention to finishing and detailing. But buy cheap, look cheap. So here's a shopping list to take with you when you go. (You can pass it on to the mortician when you're done with it.)

Shirt Notes

■ Shirts should have seven buttons (eight for tall men) in front and two or three buttons sewn inside as extras.

■ The collar should fit snugly when you button the top button, but don't do a Dangerfield: It shouldn't be so tight that you can't get a finger to fit comfortably between the collar and your neck.

■ The body of the shirt should have no more material than is necessary for a man to sit comfortably. Most of us can do without additional bulges in the middle regions, thank you.

■ The shirt should hang at least six inches below the waist. That untucked look may have been cool back when you were in prep school, but it looks cool no longer, old sport.

■ Next, the placket. This is the extra piece of material on the front of the shirt where the buttonholes go. In a quality shirt, it will be 1½ inches wide. It should also lie flat and not show any wrinkling or gathering at the seams. If the shirt fits properly, there will be no gaps between-buttons. If you want to look like you really know what you're doing, bring a ruler and count off the stitches on a one-inch seam of the placket. Fourteen stitches per inch is a sign of quality. Fewer than 11 signals low-grade goods. As for the buttonholes, examine the stitching. Avoid ragged ones with loose threads. Pull on the buttons to be sure they are sewn securely.

■ The sleeve should be fitted exactly to your arm length, which is obtained by measuring from the center of the back of your neck to your wrist. The shirt cuff should show a full half-inch beyond the sleeve of your jacket. Forgot your jacket? A good rule of thumb is that the material ends a half-inch below the point where your thumb meets your wrist. Another rule: Bend your arm; if the cuff recedes past the wrist, the sleeve is too short. Avoid sleeves described in average sizes, such as 32/33: These fit neither size well.

■ Pockets should be neatly stitched and lie flat.

■ Fabric counts. For dress, a moderately priced cotton shirt, properly laundered and starched, will always look better than even the most expensive poly-blend job.

Pants Notes

■ Pants cut too small will make a fat man fatter. Cut too large, they'll make a skinny man skinnier.

■ Slacks should fit so that they hang loosely, breaking only once—and ever so slightly—just above the shoe. What does this mean? The top of your shoe should be completely obscured all the way around the cuff. There's a little margin for error on the side of extra length, but not the other way around. Rule of thumb: Trousers should be long enough that your socks don't show when you walk.

■ The waist should fit you comfortably, but only at the point where God put your waist. Fashionable men move their waists up and down their bodies as if a waistline were a carousel pony. But you know, and your trousers know, there's just one place where the lifting end stops and the walking end starts. That's where your waistline is. Also, some of us can find our waistline simply by noting where we most precede ourselves.

■ The crotch of the trousers should be as high as is comfortable for what's known in the trade as a "clean" fit.

■ Pleats should lie flat. If you notice that they spread open, bite the bullet and try the next larger waist size. Likewise, the act of buttoning your pants should not make the pockets flare open.

● ●

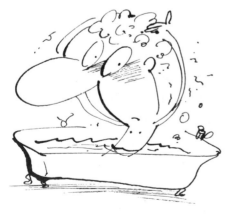

Cut Your Losses

Balding men who opt for hair transplant surgery can expect a lot of those relocated strands to go down the drain with the shampoo suds, says Henry Roenigk, M.D., dermatology department chairman at Northwestern University Medical School. But here's hope for better yields: His recent studies show that minoxidil, the hair growth drug, stabilizes hair loss after hair transplants. When ten men applied 2 percent minoxidil to the surgery site for several weeks before and after hair transplants, they lost only 20 percent of the transplanted hairs, compared with the more typical 50 percent loss for a group of men who didn't get the drug.

▪ Cuffs are optional for tall men, but they can make short men look shorter by producing a visible border between slacks and shoes.

Suit Notes

Jackets can be showcases for bad tailoring. And no other garment can make or break a man like a suit. So combine the stuff on slacks above with the stuff below to ensure that you're buying the right thing.

▪ When you try on a jacket, make sure you have all the things in your pockets you normally carry, including wallet and keys.

▪ When your arms are relaxed at your side, the back should lie perfectly flat, with no ripples and no bulging between the shoulder blades or under the arms. Likewise, the lapels should lie flat on the chest. Most important of all, be sure the collar lies flat. If it stands away from your neck, either we're talking alterations or we're talking image problem.

▪ The material in the rear of the jacket should cover your rear. While we're on the subject, a double-vented jacket generally covers it best whether you're standing or sitting. If you are extra wide, though, a single vent provides better camouflage.

▪ The sleeve should end where your wrist meets your hand. By the way, short men have almost no leeway for size, since a jacket that is too long, short, big or little will have a disastrous effect.

▪ Five signs of a cheap suit:

1. The seam down the middle of the jacket's back is a sea of little ripples extending from the neck to the center flap.

2. The pattern or weave doesn't match where two pieces of fabric meet on the back or at the sleeve.

3. The lapel intrudes on the topmost button closure.

4. The stitching around the shoulder is clearly visible.

5. The price is too good to be true.

Foot Notes

Shoes shouldn't be the first thing somebody notices about you. Shop carefully for shoes, examining all the obvious construction points.

■ Shoes should have leather uppers, or you'll be standing in sweat all day. Plastic uppers make for smelly feet, too.

■ Also, avoid shoes that feature large chunks of metal, unless you're a mountaineer, a second baseman or a lineman for the county.

■ Conventional lace-ups have five or six pairs of holes. Fewer, and you have leisure shoes. More, and you have high-tops.

■ Loafers, strictly speaking, are not appropriate for conservative business dress. If you're going to try them, tassel loafers are you're safest bet.

■ Examine the way the sole is attached to the upper: If there is no stitching, the sole is glued on. That's bad, since it's not likely the shoe can be fixed if you wear a hole in the sole. If the stitching is on the inside, many shoe repair shops will be unable to do a resole job, since the machinery for inside stitching is more expensive to buy and more difficult to operate. Also, resoling a shoe with inside stitching is more likely to alter the shoe's size. The best choice is a shoe with stitching along the outside of the upper where it meets the sole, since these shoes can be repaired easily and cheaply.

■ Leather soles present the thinnest profile and are thus best for dress shoes. Besides, leather breathes and molds beautifully to the shape of your foot.

■ Three important rules for shoe maintenance:

1. Use a shoe tree. Used faithfully, it will add a decade or so to the life of an average shoe.

2. Never wear the same pair of shoes two days in a row. Giving them a rest prevents moisture buildup and allows the leather to regain its shape. If you get them wet, stuff the toes with newspaper when you get home and keep them away from radiators.

3. Shine them. A good shoe polish or a saddle soap reinvigorates natural oils and preserves leather.

■ Socks should fit. None of that one-size-fits-you-or-your-mom stuff. Also, they should be tall enough that you never show any bare leg when you sit down.

THE SIMPLE RULE OF HATS

You can look as good as gold from the neck down, but if you top it all off with a stupid hat, you become a party joke. So when you choose a hat, use your head.

Round heads need a high-rise crown and narrow brim. Eggheads need a low crown and wide brim. Square heads should look for a medium brim with a soft crown. You long, lean, horse-faced guys need a brim about the size of Granny's front porch.

No other single piece of apparel exerts such a strong primal pull on a normal man as a cowboy hat. When a guy puts on a cowboy hat, he usually sees the back-projected movie of his mind and not the dork everyone else sees. The truth is, when guys go west for hats, they leave their brain someplace east of the Mississip. Here's what to keep on your mind when your feet are in the stirrups but your ass is on the ground.

■ Long-headed men are the only men who can successfully wear a genuine ten-gallon Stetson.

■ Round heads should go for Stetson's Flat Crown hat, first made from 1880 to 1910. Stetson took a ten-gallon hat, flattened the crown and added a slight roll-in, then shaped the brim a bit on both sides. Nice hat, provided there's no wind, since the flat crown precludes a snug, secure fit. Wild Bill wore this one on TV.

■ Oval-shaped and square heads will look best in the cowboy hat first popularized in the movies in 1935 and most often seen today. Roy and Gene wore this model. The crown is low, and the brim has both sides turned up—in theory, so it won't blow off when your horse is at a full gallop.

UNIFORMS

Lawyers don't dress like plumbers, and plumbers don't dress like foresters. Everybody's got a uniform, a profession-specific wardrobe that announces, with some precision, who he is, what he does and how much he makes doing it.

When we stop wearing our own uniform and start wearing somebody else's, we usually end up in trouble or in disguise. Either way, uniforms are a compelling notion; everybody has a closet desire to dress up as something bigger than life. You put on the right suit, and presto! Appearance becomes reality. For example, which urologist are you going to choose: The guy in the overalls marked "Bill's Septic" or the fellow clad in medic white?

—Brian Hennesey

Miracle Dentistry

It used to be that when you reached a certain age, you started losing teeth. That's changing. Let's just say the future does not look bright for denture makers.

• • • • • • • • • • • • • • • • • •

I HAVE AN UNCLE-IN-LAW whose favorite game during family reunions is to scare the bejeebers out of little kids by jutting out his dentures and clicking the china choppers in their faces. I'm not sure I understand why he finds this so funny, but I think I do know why the kids find it so scary. Whatever your age, seeing teeth anyplace but where they belong—firmly rooted in the mouth—is disquieting.

What's doubly disturbing to me about this guy is that he's saddled with false teeth while still fairly young—early 50s—and, according to my wife, he's had these choppers since *she* was a kid.

For a long time I consoled myself with the argument that his generation knew less about dental care when they were growing up and were consequently more likely to suffer tooth loss later on. It could never happen to me; I haven't had a cavity in years.

But dental experts now tell me I have no cause to be

smug, at least not just yet. Statistics show that 17 out of 100 working men still suffer the loss of more than seven teeth by age 64. Many of those cases have nothing at all to do with cavities.

Cavities are mostly a problem during childhood, when we tend to eat sweets more and care for our teeth less. Gum disease, however, is the most prevalent adult dental affliction of our time and the leading cause of tooth loss. It occurs when bacteria under the gum line create hollows or pockets that weaken the tooth's grip on the jaw. Eventually, the tooth loosens and may fall out.

MEN SUFFER MORE

According to the American Academy of Periodontology, 75 percent of adults have gum disease (more properly called periodontal disease), and three out of five who suffer from its most severe form are men. Mind you, it's not that children are exempt from gum disease. It's just that it takes years for bacteria to get under the gum line and destroy a tooth's supporting structure. So a child with gum disease may not see any signs of damage until he's well into his 30s.

But tooth loss isn't inevitable. Regular brushing and flossing can go a long way toward controlling the bacteria-bearing plaque that's at the heart of the problem. Flossing is particularly important because it removes plaque from tooth surfaces below the gum, discouraging bacteria from taking hold there. Beyond that, however, a new arsenal of tooth-saving techniques promises for the first time to actually repair damage that's already been done to teeth, gums, roots and bone. Which is to say that denture-clacking relatives may soon become a thing of the past.

Some of these advances are already in use. Perhaps the most important of them is a technique that heals weakened bones and ligaments that anchor teeth to the jaw. This is radical because in the past, dentists considered any loss of tooth-supporting structure to be irreversible.

To eradicate the hard-to-reach bacteria lodged in pockets in the gums, a periodontist makes an incision in the dental pocket, peeling back the gum like an envelope flap. He

• •

THE DAILY GRIND

Doctors have warned us that chronic stress can lead to a variety of ills ranging from headaches to heart attacks. Now dentists want to get in on the act. They report that a high-stress lifestyle can lead to tooth loss. "Stress reduces salivary flow and can weaken the body's defenses, allowing bacteria to flourish in the mouth," says Boston-area immunologist Myrin Borysenko, Ph.D. Once the bacteria penetrate the gum line, they can cause the gums to become inflamed, bleed or recede, all which can loosen teeth.

Stress can also lead to habitual grinding of the teeth, a condition known as bruxism. This actually wears down tooth surfaces and can expose and irritate the nerve inside the tooth. Once that happens, you may need root canal surgery.

If you have dental trouble, should you try to relax more? Absolutely, say the experts. Just don't consider it a substitute for regular brushing and flossing and dental checkups.

• •

cleans the root surface thoroughly and then places a swatch of Gore-Tex material over the damaged area. When the flap is sutured up, the material keeps gum tissue away from the roots and bone, boosting their natural healing powers and encouraging damaged parts to grow back. "Already, teeth that we once deemed hopeless can be saved," says John Dmytryk, D.M.D., Ph.D., assistant professor at the University of Oklahoma College of Dentistry.

The only problem with the procedure is that a second surgery is normally needed to remove the Gore-Tex. Dr. Dmytryk and his colleagues are now experimenting with materials that dissolve harmlessly in the body, making the second operation unnecessary. They should be available within two years.

Periodontists are further able to boost bone regrowth by packing pulverized bone crystals around the tooth root. The material fuses with the jaw, speeding the rebuilding process. A few years down the road, doctors may be able to simply apply synthetic versions of the body's own growth-stimulating hormones to the roots of teeth, encouraging the body to make its own dental repairs.

ANTIBIOTIC WEAPONS

With any luck, however, you'll never need surgery at all, thanks to new ways of fighting gum-ravaging bacteria with drugs.

One experimental method is to wrap at-risk teeth with fibers that slowly release concentrated doses of antibiotic. Another is to inject the medicine directly into the gum pockets where bacteria are growing. These new treatments are better than already-available antibiotics that you swallow because they hit bacteria with stronger doses of medicine without producing side effects such as upset stomach. Both new techniques are awaiting approval from the Food and Drug Administration (FDA).

Researchers are also experimentally using the drug flurbiprofen, an anti-inflammatory agent that's a relative of the painkiller ibuprofen, to strengthen the jawbone against bacterial attacks. Flurbiprofen blocks the formation of substances released by the body that trigger bone erosion. Some early studies suggest that once you have periodontal disease, daily doses of this drug will make you resistant to any further damage from bacteria, says Sebastian G. Ciancio, D.D.S., chairman of the periodontology department at the State University of New York at Buffalo. The FDA hasn't yet approved flurbiprofen for these purposes. More clinical studies are needed before the FDA okays its prescription for gum disease patients.

NEW DIAGNOSTIC TOOLS

None of these new developments will help you unless you know you have a problem, making advances in diagnosis just as important as those in treatment. "We're talking about a chronic disease that has to be monitored constantly," says William Clark, D.D.S., D.M.S.C., director of the Periodontal Disease Research Center at the University of Florida College of Dentistry. "The more you know about what's going on, the better your therapy will be."

Already in use are new tools that make the normally tedious and unpleasant pocket-measuring exam faster and more accurate. One such device is a probe that's linked to a computer, so it records the depths of the dental pockets automatically, instantly comparing the results with previous readings. Other computerized equipment avoids the use of a probe entirely by comparing x-rays taken at different times and pointing up tiny differences between the images. Both offer an early warning of a developing problem.

Researchers have also come up with better, easier ways to identify decay-causing bacteria. They can spot potential problems in a dental pocket by checking for changes in temperature, enzyme activity and even the DNA of plaque below the gum line.

What about the tooth that's healthy below the gum line but that has been broken or cracked from, say, a sports injury? There are advances to report here, too.

For years, the best way to repair a broken tooth was to affix a protective cap of metal or porcelain, a procedure that required the dentist to drill away a substantial portion of real tooth to make room for the replacement material. Now

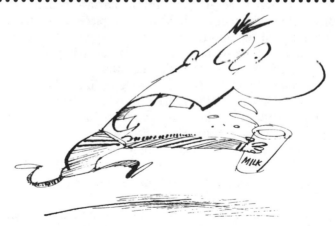

Tooth CPR

Should you ever lose a tooth in an accident, it will begin to die within 15 minutes. But you can buy a few hours time to get to a dentist by plopping the tooth in a container of cold milk.

eggshell-thin veneers can be bonded to the tooth by drilling away only a small amount of the enamel. Before getting a tooth capped, it's a good idea to ask your dentist if a veneer might be appropriate. Veneers require no anesthesia and are kinder to gum tissue and cheaper than caps. The best are made from porcelain, which resists stains better than real enamel. (Expect to pay about $400 to $800 for a veneer, $500 to $1,000 for a cap.)

MIRACLE IMPLANTS

Finally, a word must be said about what to do if you actually lose teeth. The biggest news here is dental implants, which now make it possible to have a mouthful of false teeth that are just as stable as the real kind. Implants are lightweight metal cylinders or blades that substitute for natural roots and provide a firm anchor for your false teeth. Some are surgically set into the jawbone. Others are inserted under the gum tissue to fit snugly over jaw crevices and undercuts.

There are a number of benefits to implants. First, if you're replacing a single tooth, you can avoid getting a bridge. Bridges are artificial teeth that are cemented to adjoining healthy teeth to hold them in place. Bridging is a time-honored technique but one that inevitably requires some paring of the supporting teeth. Because implants stand alone, neighboring teeth remain unscathed.

Second, if you've lost a lot of teeth, implants can help you avoid conventional dentures. Firmly anchoring four to six false teeth in the jaw with implants provides a stable structure to which neighboring fakes can be attached.

Even if you already have removable dentures, you can benefit from this new technology. There's an implant-based snap-type attachment that can keep your choppers more solidly in place.

Sorry to say, not everyone who's lost a tooth is a candidate for jawbone-based implants. If the bone is too shallow or porous, it may not provide enough of a footing for the standard cylinder or blade implant. But even if that's so, ask your dentist about the over-the-bone kind.

TWO-STEP PROCESS

Installing implants usually takes two steps about four to six months apart. First, the implant is put in and allowed to fuse with the bone; later, the tooth is attached. Costs range from $1,000 to $2,000 for the implant alone. Add to that the cost for diagnostic work, the false tooth itself and any follow-up care. The fees are not currently covered by dental plans, but that's expected to change as early as this year.

For information on doctors in your area who offer these new techniques, send a self-addressed, stamped business-size envelope to the American Academy of Periodontology's referral service at 737 North Michigan Avenue, Suite 800, Department MH, Chicago, IL 60611.

Experts are quick to point out that prevention with brushing and flossing is still the best way to keep your teeth healthy and attractive. But with all these new developments at hand, Dr. Ciancio has one further bit of advice: "Don't invest in denture companies."

—Richard Allan

Part 8

BOD LIKE A ROCK

Build Bulk Fast

*You can grow muscles quicker than
you ever thought. Here are the ten secrets
of quick strength.*

• • • • • • • • • • • • • • • • • • •

YOU EAT RIGHT. You stick to your workout program. You can climb three flights of stairs without needing an oxygen tank. You're in good shape, and you know it. But you want more: You want everybody *else* to know it.

Let's face it, nobody is impressed by your cardiovascular fitness. What you need are some muscles to go with your healthy heart and lungs. And the good news is that you can get them—fast.

Any kind of weight work is going to make you stronger than you were before you started out, but the wrong kind of routine—one aimed at endurance, for example—isn't going to build up muscle as fast or as much. If pure strength is what you're after, you need to design your routine according to specific power-pumping principles.

This is not, by the way, a misplaced priority. It's a fact that if you look like a god, with muscles like marble, you'll feel better, have more energy and probably live longer as well.

With all this in mind, we asked experts in both exercise physiology and strength training to explain the secrets of fast muscle growth. To look like a god, they say, you have to follow some basic commandments. What you stand to gain is six to nine pounds of pure new muscle in six months. "That's a lot," says Wayne Westcott, Ph.D., YMCA national strength-training consultant. "You'll look firmer, fitter, more toned and less flabby, with greater build, particularly in the chest, thighs, shoulders and back." Having all that is about as close to being a god as most of us can hope to get.

Work big muscles before small ones. Big areas of the body such as the legs, chest, back and shoulders are not single muscles but *groups* of muscles, and these should be attacked first, for two reasons.

One, this method is efficient, since you attack many muscles at once. A leg press, for example, simultaneously works the quadriceps, hamstrings, buttocks and calves. Upper body examples of good big-muscle exercises (also known as compound exercises) are the bench press and military press.

Two, compound exercises don't wear you out as fast. "Let's say you do a triceps pushdown—a single-muscle exercise—before you do a bench press," explains Dr. Westcott. "You need the triceps to do the bench press, and if they're already fatigued, it'll weaken the effort you're putting into the big muscles." If you're doing less work where it really counts, you're not getting strong as fast as you could.

If you're pressed for time, you can get a decent workout that hits all the major muscle groups in about a half-hour with only six exercises: squat, upright row, bench press, military press, pull-down and crunch. (See the box on page 205 for directions.)

Lift heavy weights. Working with the heaviest weights you can handle for 8 to 15 repetitions builds muscle fastest, the experts say. By contrast, the popular circuit-training method of using higher repetitions and lighter weights is geared toward building your endurance, not your strength, says Michael H. Stone, Ph.D., professor of exercise science at Appalachian State University. Weights build strength by putting strain on the muscles and actually breaking them down. It's the recovery—the "healing" of this breakdown—that makes muscles bigger and tougher. Lifting heavy weights makes this process happen more quickly.

The question is, how heavy is heavy? The American College of Sports Medicine and the national YMCA advise working with weights heavy enough to make your muscles give out after 60 to 90 seconds of steady lifting. Done properly, each lift should take about 7 seconds, which gives you 8 to 12 repetitions.

That doesn't mean you should pile on the metal plates when you first get started in a lifting program. On the contrary, Dr. Westcott recommends that during your first week you start off with lighter weights to get your body conditioned for heavier work. For example, use a weight you can lift comfortably 12 times. During the second week, add enough weight to make 12 repetitions difficult. During the third week, add weight to make 9 or 10 repetitions difficult. "That's right where you want to be," he says. "Stay there until you can do 12 comfortably, then add five pounds."

Always add weight gradually. As a rule of thumb, never add more than 5 percent of the weight you're already lifting.

Do three sets in succession. For example, if you're planning on doing three sets of bench presses, do all three before moving on to the next exercise. Again, this approach differs from circuit training, where you do one rapid set, then move on to the next exercise. "There's nothing wrong with doing circuits per se, but they're a poor way to get strong," says Dr. Stone. Why? Because they violate commandment number one. They fatigue all the body's muscles before you have a chance to really challenge each big muscle group. As a general rule, shoot for three sets of each exercise before moving on. Studies show that doing three

THE 30-MINUTE POWER WORKOUT

When time is tight, do these six exercises to target your body's big muscle groups. To avoid muscle pulls, remember to warm up with a few minutes of jogging or calisthenics before lifting.

Squats. In a standing position, grip a barbell with hands shoulder-width apart. Lift the weight over your head, then slowly lower it behind your head until it rests on your shoulders. Now squat down as if sitting on a chair until your thighs are parallel with the floor. Then press up to the starting position. Repeat.

Upright rows. Grasp the middle of a barbell with your hands about six inches apart. Standing with your back straight, raise the bar up to your chin, pause a second, then slowly lower the weight. Repeat.

Bench presses. Lie on an exercise bench with your feet flat on the floor. Grasp the barbell with your hands slightly wider than shoulder-width apart. Lift the bar off the rack and slowly lower it to your chest. Then press the weight up until you can lock your elbows. Keep your hips on the bench at all times. Repeat.

Military presses. Sit on an exercise bench and grasp a barbell with your hands shoulder-width apart. Lift the weight over your head and rest it on the back of your shoulders, then press it up until your arms are fully extended. Slowly lower the weight back to your shoulders. Repeat.

Pulldowns. To do this exercise, you need a lat machine on a multistation gym. Stand facing the lat machine, reach up, and take an overhand grip on the bar with your hands three to five inches wider than your shoulders. Straighten your arms and use your weight to pull your body downward until you can kneel. (Some machines have a seat on which to sit and a padded restraint you can wedge your knees under.) Now use your upper back and arms to pull the bar down to touch behind your neck. Hold for a count of one, then return slowly to the starting position. Repeat.

Crunches. Lie on your back with your knees bent. Cross your arms over your chest. Tighten your abdominals, press your chin into your chest, and curl up until your shoulders leave the floor. Hold for a count of one, then return to the mat. Repeat.

sets delivers the biggest rewards; after three, the benefits sharply taper off.

Be smooth. When exercising with weights, slow and smooth is better than fast and jerky. Rapid movements with heavy weights put tremendous stress on both muscles and tendons, Dr. Westcott says. There's nothing like being side-lined with a muscle tear to keep you from getting strong. Also, slow exercising ensures that you're not "cheating"—that neither gravity nor momentum is doing any of the work for you.

Break down, then take a break. Because strength training is equal parts breakdown and recovery, it's vital that you give your muscles enough of a rest between bouts of exercise. This applies both to the time between visits to the gym and to the time between sets during the workout.

To get strong fast, you need to take fairly long breathers between sets: two to four minutes, according to certified strength and conditioning specialist Ken Kontor, president of Conditioning Press in Lincoln, Nebraska. Cooling your jets on a bench may feel like a waste of time, Kontor says, but while you're idling, your energy tanks are being refilled. You'll be able to handle heavier weights, which means you'll get faster gains.

As for between-workout time, give yourself a day of rest—two if you're just starting your program. If you want to lift every day, do only upper body exercises one day, lower body the next.

Mix machines and free weights. Both types of equipment offer distinct advantages, and a program that includes both is better than a program that makes use of only one. Machines do a better job of guiding specific muscles through a full range of motion, so you call upon the entire muscle during a given exercise. This is particularly important on exercises that take the muscle through an arc, such as leg and arm curls, or on flies that pump up the chest.

Dumbbells and barbells, by pulling into play the muscles needed for balance, build whole muscle groups and therefore help create bulk. They also build more tendon and ligament strength. Have an instructor show you proper form on all free-weight exercises.

Make the easy part hard. There are two parts to

every exercise: lifting the weight and lowering it again. It's sensible to assume that most muscle building comes from lifting, because it seems more difficult. But studies find that the lowering, or "negative," phase may be more important. According to sports medicine specialist Lyle Micheli, M.D., of Harvard Medical School, exercises consisting solely of the negative phase can build muscle as much as 20 percent faster than positive-only exercises. To do a negative-only bench press, for example, you would slowly lower a barbell loaded with extra-heavy weight to your chest, then have spotters lift it back up for you. But you can get nearly the same benefits simply by slowing your motion on the down-swing. Concentrate on slower, better-controlled negative movements. As a guide, the experts advise spending two seconds lifting and four seconds lowering.

● ●

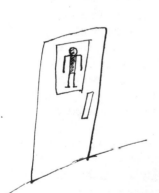
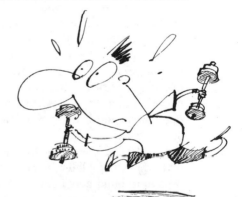

Ex-Lax with Weights

New research suggests strength training may accelerate the time it takes for food to move through the body by as much as 56 percent. Because other studies have indicated that slow movement of food through the body may play a role in colon cancer development, strength training could be one way to reduce that cancer risk. Why pumping iron helps is a mystery, according to Ben F. Hurley, Ph.D., director of the Exercise Science Lab at the University of Maryland College of Health and Human Performance. It may have to do with strength training's effects on chemicals involved in digestion.

Be dedicated—for six months. The biggest gains from weight training come almost immediately, within the first three to six months. "We all have a certain genetic potential for strength," says Peter Lemon, Ph.D., professor of applied physiology at Kent State University. "If you exercise three times a week for several months, you'll already have realized most of that potential, and your gains from then on will be minimal." After six months, you can slack off: Dr. Lemon says you can maintain those early gains by working out as little as once a week.

Still, some men want to continue gaining even after they reach the six-month plateau. To do it, you need to vary your routine, adding new exercises that either target new muscles or stimulate the same ones in different ways. "The professional bodybuilders refer to this as 'sculpting,' " Kontor says. Here's one way to do it: Let's say you do bench presses and military presses on Mondays, Wednesdays and Fridays. On Wednesdays, instead of doing regular bench presses, do presses on an inclined or declined bench. In place of doing military presses with a barbell as usual, use dumbbells, alternating each hand, or do lateral shoulder raises. The new exercises work the same muscle groups, but they do so at slightly different angles, which strengthens any underdeveloped areas and keeps you growing. For more guidance, consult a trainer.

Eat more. First, it's time to debunk the long-standing myth that weight lifters need to eat more protein. True, it takes protein to build new muscle, and your body uses a little more of the stuff when you are weight training. However, most of us are already taking in 50 to 100 percent more protein from our diets than we need. "Most of the extra we get either is burned off or turns to fat," says Dr. Micheli. "Adding more to your diet won't hinder you, but it won't help, either."

Instead, experts say, you need to get more *energy* from food. "The main problem weight lifters have, particularly men, is that they don't get enough calories," says Susan Kleiner, Ph.D., R.D., nutritional consultant to the Cleveland Browns. Putting on muscle raises your metabolism, which makes the body burn fuel faster. If your calorie intake falls behind your body's demands for energy, you won't be able to work out as hard as you need to. Experts say that an average man of, say, 155 pounds who normally consumes about 2,400 calories per day should get at least 900 more calories per day when weight training.

At least 60 percent of these added calories should come from carbohydrates, which is the highest-octane form of fuel your body can get. You'll get about 900 calories from carbohydrates by eating two cups of pasta with tomato sauce, two pieces of bread and a glass of fruit juice. "That's like a whole extra meal," says Gail Butterfield, Ph.D., R.D., a sports nutritionist and director of nutrition studies at the Veterans Affairs Medical Center in Palo Alto, California. If you can't spare the time for an extra meal in your day, you can generally make up the slack by taking extra helpings of carbohydrate-rich foods such as pasta, rice, beans, breads and cereals at regular meals.

Be selective about supplements. Most pills and powders touted as muscle-building aids have little value. But a few minerals really do offer a benefit. For example, a new study at Western Washington University suggests that taking magnesium may double your strength gains when used during a resistance-training routine.

In the study, a group of 13 people with low dietary magnesium who took magnesium supplements during a seven-week exercise program of leg extensions and presses recorded a 20 percent increase in leg strength—twice that of a low-magnesium group that took placebos while doing the same program. The average amount of magnesium used in the study was 500 milligrams from both diet and supplements, nearly 1.5 times the Recommended Dietary Allowance (RDA). "Most of the population gets well below the RDA," says Lorraine Brilla, Ph.D., of the university's exercise and sport science laboratory. You can make sure your muscles are well supplied with the mineral by eating nuts, dark green vegetables, bananas and whole grains.

Some evidence suggests it may also be useful to get more zinc and copper, both of which are lost in sweat during exercise. Zinc and copper are found in abundance in milk, beans, fortified breakfast cereals and beef.

—Richard Laliberte

Excuse Busters

*How to stick to your workout on days when
excuses come easier than exercises.*

• • • • • • • • • • • • • • • • • •

REMEMBER THAT PLEDGE YOU MADE last January?
Somewhere amid the sound of champagne corks popping
and the whistles and bells of New Year's Eve, you said it—
maybe out loud, maybe just to yourself. It went something
like "I will go jogging every other morning," or maybe it
was "I'm gonna hit the gym each day after work." Maybe it
was something more simple, a general "I'm going to get
back in shape."

And you did. Or started to. But then things got crazy at
work, and there were two dinner parties that you *had* to
show up at, and you missed a workout, and then a day off
turned into a week, and next thing you knew you were back
on the couch with a blister on your remote control thumb.

Well, don't be too hard on yourself. Studies show that
50 percent of people drop out of their exercise programs
within six months. But on days when excuses come easier
than exercises, there are a number of tactics you can use to
help you stick to your fitness routine. So renew your vows.
Here's how you can get in shape and stay that way.

First, the experts say, it's essential to set a *short-term*
goal for yourself. "Most people start with a six-month or
yearlong vision, but that vision can be lost pretty quickly
when you're feeling run-down," says Dave Scott, professional triathlete and six-time winner of the Ironman competition. Instead, set a two-week short-term goal, and make it
specific. If your long-term plan is to get a 32-inch waist, for
example, figure out a specific way to get it (say, running
three times a week), and then make it your goal to simply
get out there three times.

A second key tactic is to recruit a workout partner. You
can compare goals and provide each other with a little
encouragement and friendly competition. Just as important,
you'll have someone to answer to if you start to slack off.

"This is useful for those bad mornings when you don't feel like rolling out of bed," says Wayne Westcott, Ph.D., national strength-training consultant for the YMCA.

Here are some other stick-to-it tips from leading trainers around the country.

Put your money where your muscle is. A study at Michigan State University found that people who bet $40 that they could stick with their program for six months had a 97 percent success rate. Less than 20 percent of those who didn't take the bet were able to stick to their routines. Bet a workout partner that the first man to slack off pays up. Hell, bet a cool grand, and you'll never miss a workout again.

Count backward. When you're counting repetitions, start with your target number and count backward, says Pat Croce, physical conditioning coach for Philadelphia's Flyers and 76ers. When you get toward the end of your set, you'll be thinking how few you have left instead of how many you've done.

Get a periodic fitness test. Most YMCAs and many health clubs offer fitness testing, says Dr. Westcott. Testing your body composition, strength or cardiovascular fitness on a regular basis can give you tangible proof that your workout is working. You can probably see that in the mirror, but it's good to have it on paper.

Get your log rolling. For most of us, keeping a training log ranks alongside changing the baby's diapers on the interest scale. Still, we do change diapers (sometimes), and the experts say that we should log our fitness progress as well. If ordinary pencil-and-paper bookkeeping bores you, get high-tech. These computer programs do some of the work for you.

■ The Athlete's Log from B & B Software, Inc., P.O. Box 10212, Eugene, OR 97440. Tracks your progress in running, swimming, biking and a variety of other activities; about $50.

■ Ultra Coach from Flite Controls, (800) 729-1908. Lets you tailor a six-week running, swimming or biking schedule to your fitness level; about $60.

Slot your race. A common mistake men make is to first decide that they'll run five miles a day, *then* try to find time to do it. Instead, pick the time slot first. If you know you can clear out 40 minutes at lunchtime three times a week, you'll be able to realistically pick a type of exercise

YOU ARE NOT EXCUSED

Creativity is a wonderful thing, but applying your imaginative powers to avoiding your workout is not productive. Instead, try some of these answers to some typical slacker excuses.

IT'S TOO DAMNED COLD OUT

- Smear petroleum jelly on your nostrils, lips and face before you go out. It will help prevent freezing and wind-burn.

- When you're cycling or running, start out with the wind behind you and return facing the wind. This way you get a boost when you're cold. Wind in your face is more tolerable once you've warmed up.

- To deal with a runny nose, wear washable terry-cloth wrist-bands. You know what to do with them.

- Wear a hat. Forty percent of body heat escapes through an uncovered head.

- Look for cover. Tree-lined streets and wooded trails are always much warmer than wide-open roads where the wind can build up.

IT'S TOO DAMNED HOT OUT

- Drink six to eight ounces of fluids for every 15 minutes of exercise in heat. Your body relies on sweating to cool itself. Try sticking a three-quarters-full water bottle in the freezer the night before. It'll thaw out slowly, giving you cool sips along the way.

- Wear a headband. It will prevent the salty sweat from running down your face and stinging your eyes.

- Before exercising, dampen clothing, then wring it out. The evaporation will provide air-conditioning.

that will fit into that time constraint (say, a 20-minute run with a warm-up, stretches and a shower).

Take it easy. "One of the things we've found is that high-intensity programs tend to have a very high dropout rate," says Michael Pollock, Ph.D., director of the Center

- Wear light clothing rather than going without a shirt. Sunburn causes body temperature to increase, making you lose more fluids than normal.

- For long workouts, spread a little bit of petroleum jelly on the bottom of your feet and in between your toes. This will keep sweaty feet from blistering. Wearing acrylic socks instead of cotton ones will also reduce your risk of blisters.

IT'S RAINING/SNOWING/SLEETING/HAILING

- Keep your feet warm by dusting the inside of your socks with talcum powder (to keep them dry), then cover your socks with plastic bags.

- Look for shoes with neoprene collars—the same material they make wet suits out of. These keep feet warm even when wet.

I CAN'T GET AWAY FROM MY OFFICE

- Schedule your workout like you schedule your career. If your secretary makes appointments for your business lunches, ask her to schedule your workouts as well. When one needs to be bumped, she can reschedule it for you.

I WANT TO SPEND MORE TIME
WITH MY WIFE/KIDS/GIRLFRIEND/SCHNAUZER

- Buy a jogging stroller. You'll not only free your spouse from baby-sitting duty, you'll also be spending time with your kid that's undiluted by TV and other distractions.

- Pick an occasional workout such as biking that the family can join you in. How to break a sweat while biking with the kids? Stay in low gear on the flats, medium gear for hill climbing. Do ten push-ups against the handlebar per mile.

for Exercise Science at the University of Florida. It's far more important to be consistent in your program than to try to drain every last bit of fitness benefit from each workout.

Entertain yourself. Get some extra value out of your exercise time by reading the paper or watching the morning news on your stationary bike. Listening to a personal stereo helps pass the miles while running. Better yet, play books on tape.

Set a 20-minute rule. Make a deal with yourself that even when you're dog tired, you'll do a light workout on your scheduled days. "I have a 20-minute rule," says Scott. "Even if I only work up a light sweat or get my heart rate up to 55 to 65 percent of maximum, most of the time that's enough."

Vary the program. Nobody said your routine had to be routine. Training hard one day and easy the next is a success secret for many elite athletes. "I know that if I pushed myself hard yesterday, then I don't have to maintain that level of intensity today," says marathoner Frank Shorter, Olympic gold and silver medalist. Another way to vary your routine is to cross-train: "With cross-training, you can pick the activity you like the best on days when you really don't feel like working out," says Shorter.

Check your ego at the door. If you do it all for vanity, you might not be doing yourself very much good. In a study, researchers at the University of Texas found that those who took up exercise mainly to improve appearance experienced a *drop* in feelings of self-worth. If you want to remind yourself why it's important to stay fit, try hanging a family photo on your exercise room wall, recommends Jake Steinfeld, of ESPN's "Body by Jake." "That's the motivation for me now," Steinfeld claims. "I've got a baby daughter and a beautiful wife; I want to stick around."

Throw yourself a bone. It might seem counterproductive to reward yourself with a dinner of lobster Newburg after losing five pounds, but if that's what it will take to get you over the hump, go ahead and make reservations. Healthier choices could include a new warm-up outfit, top-of-the-line sneakers or an upgraded health club membership. Just make sure that your bonus is tied to achieving a tangible goal. Ordering a double-cheese pizza simply because you've "been pretty good lately" is a cop-out, not a reward.

Finally, if you miss a workout, don't beat yourself up over it. Acknowledge that you skipped it, figure out why, then get back on the horse. "If you miss a day, simply continue the schedule," says Dr. Westcott.

—*Stephen Perrine*

Gold Medal Advice

*Olympic coaches offer their best tips
for weekend athletes.*

• • • • • • • • • • • • • • • • • •

IN THE OLYMPICS, THE DIFFERENCE between the three guys who get to stand up on the platform with medals around their necks and the ones who have to watch them from the sidelines is often so slight it can be measured in hundredths of a second. Olympic skills are honed to their sharpest not just through practice but by understanding *how* to win. "Being a good athlete isn't enough anymore; you also have to keep up with the latest advances in sports training," says Tom Crawford, director of the U.S. Olympic Committee's Coaching Development Program.

Enter the coach, whose duties range from high-tech to low-tech, from scouring sports medicine journals for new ideas to offering a simple word of encouragement at just the right moment. Any athlete who is serious about his sport can benefit from this kind of support. To help you reach for your own personal best, we went to our nation's top Olympic coaches and asked them a simple question: What single factor makes the most difference to the success of an athletic program? Their answers are fundamental, insightful, motivating. Here's what they had to say.

TOM TELLEZ, PERSONAL COACH FOR OLYMPIC GOLD MEDALIST CARL LEWIS

Run your own race. "At the start of the 100-meter dash in the 1988 Olympics in Seoul, Ben Johnson broke out of the blocks very fast. Carl caught a glimpse of him out of the corner of his eye and tried to go with him. Although he came in right behind Johnson, I think he could have run faster, and maybe even won, if he had stuck to the race plan we worked on in practice. Many times an athlete's zeal for competition actually hinders his performance. For the best results, athletes have to practice the way they want to compete and compete the way they practice.

"This logic doesn't apply only to elite athletes. You should always make a plan for meet day and stick with it."

EDDIE REESE, HEAD COACH, MEN'S U.S. OLYMPIC SWIM TEAM

Cut yourself some slack time. "After a hard workout, cut back and give your body time to recover. Slow down a little and don't feel guilty about it. Studies have shown that athletes who consistently push themselves too hard don't perform as well as those who know when to ease off a bit."

DRAGOMIR CIOROSLAN, RESIDENT WEIGHT-LIFTING COACH AT THE OLYMPIC TRAINING CENTER, COLORADO SPRINGS, COLORADO

Steady yourself. "Getting to the gym on a regular basis is the most important thing a weight lifter can do. If you're serious about building your body, you need to hit the weights at least twice a week. You'll get more benefit from doing a little every week than you will from doing too much one week and nothing the next. In addition, to get the most out of your strength-training program, you need to throw in some aerobic exercise like running or biking two or three times a week. Shaping up your cardiovascular system will give you the endurance to keep your intensity up throughout your strength workouts."

CHUCK DALY, HEAD COACH, U.S. OLYMPIC BASKETBALL TEAM

Program your success. "At the professional or Olympic level, there are lots of guys with plenty of talent but who lack the motivation to work hard. Although motivation is partly internal, it can be developed. The best way to do this is through peer pressure. Playing next to, or against, someone who is highly motivated is an inspiring experience.

"If your workout program is in a rut, try working out with a friend who's more dedicated. Chances are some of his motivation and enthusiasm will rub off."

YVES AURIOL, COACH, U.S. OLYMPIC FENCING TEAM

Work on your mental mettle. "For most sports, mental conditioning is as important as physical conditioning. Taking a minute to tell yourself you're doing a good job builds confidence and motivation, and this enables you to work much harder than if you're constantly criticizing your effort. Even when you're having a bad day, look for something you're doing right and praise yourself for it."

JOE BYRD, HEAD COACH, U.S. OLYMPIC BOXING TEAM

Sting like a butterfly, eat like a horse. "The month before an international competition, one of my fighters dropped 20 pounds to get to a lower weight class where he thought he'd have a better chance of winning a medal. He lost the weight but got creamed in the first match. He just didn't have the stamina to go all out for three rounds.

"In order to maximize their strength, endurance, energy and reflexes, athletes in training need to eat at least three medium-size meals (600 to 1,000 calories each) a day, with plenty of high-carbohydrate snacks such as fruits, bread or cereal in between. Those who go hungry simply don't have what it takes to make it through intense workouts."

LOTHAR OSIANDER, HEAD COACH, U.S. OLYMPIC SOCCER TEAM

Nail boredom. "Whenever we play several tournaments in a row, my guys have a hard time generating the intensity they need to play their best. Instead of yelling at these guys to work harder, I usually tell them to take a few days off, or I change their routine. For example, we'll get off the soccer field and go play basketball for a day or two. They're still developing team skills and fitness, but they're able to work harder, since they're not bored. And it doesn't take long before they're itching to get back on the field.

"If you've been doing the same workout for several weeks or months and you're finding it more and more difficult to get to the gym or to get through your workout, chances are you could benefit from doing something totally different."

ERV HUNT, ASSISTANT COACH, U.S. OLYMPIC TRACK AND FIELD TEAM

See the big picture. "In order to get the most out of your exercise program, you need to balance the stresses in your life. If you're having a tough week at work, for example, it's best to keep your workouts light. Don't skip workouts; just don't go all out. Do two sets instead of three, run with a slower partner, or work on your form—anything to keep the blood flowing.

"On the other hand, if things are looking especially clear for you on the job, work out for an extra 15 to 30 minutes or raise your intensity slightly."

ALADAR KOGLER, PH.D., COACH, U.S. OLYMPIC FENCING TEAM; SPORT PSYCHOLOGIST, U.S. NATIONAL TEAM

Learn to focus. "When my athletes come into the gym, they have a million things on their mind—work, school, family, practically everything except fencing. But like any job, in order for them to maximize their time investment, they have to temporarily eliminate distractions and focus on the task at hand. Even if they're just running, they need to be aware of their form and the amount of effort they're putting into it.

"Before every practice, I have my athletes do 15 to 20 minutes of yoga-type stretching in which they pay special attention to their breathing. The stretching keeps their muscles flexible, and listening to their own breathing forces them to concentrate and relax. Believe it or not, these few minutes really make them better athletes."

BOBBY DOUGLAS, HEAD COACH, U.S. OLYMPIC FREESTYLE WRESTLING TEAM

Flex your muscles. "Like most men, my athletes hate to stretch. They'd rather be on the mat wrestling or in the weight room, where they feel like they're working out. But even though stretching doesn't get their hearts pounding and sweat flowing, it's probably the most effective way they can improve their performance. It increases their range of motion and produces a longer stride, smoother stroke or better follow-through. In addition, stretching is a great way to ward off injury. A flexible muscle is much more resistant to pulls and tears than a tight one, so by staying loose you'll lose less training time to injuries.

"Before *and* after every practice, I have my athletes do a minimum of 15 minutes of stretching."

MIKE KELLER, TRACK COACH FOR DAN O'BRIEN, AMERICAN RECORD HOLDER, DECATHLON

Ask for advice. "When Dan first started in the decathlon, he constantly trained in the events he did well in and neglected the ones that frustrated him. But to be competitive on an international level, you can't afford to have many weaknesses, so I had Dan spend more time on his weaker events, such as the discus, javelin and 1500. In fact, Dan now has two coaches. I work with him on the running events and hurdles, and Rick Sloan from Washington State University coaches his throwing and jumping. It's a great mix, and Dan gets the benefit of having two sets of eyes watch his progress. Now he's a true all-around decathlete, not to mention champion.

"The lesson applies to anyone who's serious about his sport. You should work with a coach or fitness instructor once in a while. A knowledgeable coach will not only be able to spot problems in your form; he'll also be able to take an objective look at your fitness program and tell you what you should work on, whether you need more rest and if you need to make any changes in your diet."

ED JACOBY, ASSISTANT COACH, U.S. OLYMPIC TRACK AND FIELD TEAM

Fix your form. "Many of the runners I work with have small biomechanical flaws in their stride. The most common one I see is overstriding. An overly long stride is actually less efficient than a shorter one, and it can also lead to chronic hamstring problems. At Boise State, I've had many talented runners ruin their running careers by using too long a stride.

"The problem here is that most athletes, not just runners, tend to ignore small flaws in their form, and instead, they concentrate on their endurance and intensity. This is asking for trouble. Athletes need to work on their mechanics first, and the rest will follow."

JOSE HIGUERAS, PERSONAL COACH FOR OLYMPIC TENNIS PLAYER JIM COURIER

Develop a secret weapon. "To succeed, tennis players need to master at least one stroke that they can always depend on, like a big forehand or a smashing serve. Having one deadly stroke is highly intimidating to your opponent. He doesn't dare hit to your strength, so he's more likely to stray from his normal game plan and make more errors. Jim's big forehand, which enables him to hit winners from the baseline, was probably the main reason he beat Andre Agassi in the finals of the 1991 French Open."

ANN GRANDJEAN, CHIEF NUTRITION CONSULTANT TO THE U.S. OLYMPIC COMMITTEE

Take the waters. "While exercising, athletes lose tremendous amounts of water. It's not uncommon for even a conditioned athlete to sweat away a quart per hour of exercise. Unfortunately, thirst lags far behind the body's need for fluids, making dehydration—and the cramps, heat exhaustion and heatstroke that can go along with it—a real risk for athletes. To keep your performance at peak levels and reduce your risk of dehydration, drink eight ounces of water 10 minutes before a workout and continue drinking four to six ounces every 15 to 20 minutes while exercising. To top off your stores, drink at least another eight ounces within 30 minutes after exercising."

—*Dan Bensimhon*

Best Moves

We've examined 7,905,432 possible exercises.
Here are the 16 best for men.

• • • • • • • • • • • • • • • • • •

IT HAPPENS. YOU GET all geared up for an exercise program. You start off with a bang, make some quick early improvement but then seem to lose your momentum. When you haven't been making gains for a few weeks, often the problem is that the exercises you've chosen are ineffective. "There are a thousand different exercises you can do to build strength and endurance," says Bob Keating, M.D., a sports medicine fellow at Ohio Physical Therapy and Sports Medicine in Cleveland. "The problem is they're not all equal."

To get the most out of your workouts, you need to select exercises that best challenge the body's major muscle groups and work them through their entire range of motion. Following are the 16 most effective exercises you can do to build your body. Stop wasting time with the wrong exercises and get working.

Neck. Freehand neck resistance: Sit on the end of a bench with your back straight. Place your right hand over your right ear and resist with your neck muscles as you tilt your head first toward your left shoulder and then back toward your right. Do 10 to 12 repetitions, then repeat the exercise using your left hand.

Upper back. Upright rows: Standing, grip a barbell with your hands no more than six inches apart, palms down. Begin with your arms hanging down so that the weight rests against the front of your thighs. Slowly lift the weight up to your chin, keeping it close to your body all the way up. Return it to the starting position. Do 10 to 12 repetitions.

Mid-back. Wide-grip rear pulldowns: Kneeling in front of the lat pulldown section of a weight machine, reach up and grab the ends of the bar so that your hands are approximately 36 inches apart. Pull the bar down until it touches the back of your neck just above the shoulders. Return the bar to the starting position. Do 10 to 12 repetitions.

Chest. Barbell bench presses: Lie on a bench and grip a barbell with your hands slightly more than shoulder-width apart. Lift the bar so that it is directly over your breastbone. Slowly lower the weight until it just touches your chest. Then press the bar up to the starting position. Do 8 to 12 repetitions.

Sides. Dumbbell side bends: Standing with your feet shoulder-width apart, hold a dumbbell in your right hand, with your palm facing your body. With your right arm straight down at your side, place your left hand on your left hip. Keeping your back straight, slowly bend as far to the right as possible; then bend as far to the left as possible. Do 12 to 15 full repetitions. Switch the weight to the left hand and repeat.

Front thighs. Leg extensions: Sitting upright in a leg extension machine, which you'll find in most gyms, tuck your feet under the footpads. Lift the pads up with your feet until your legs are extended. Hold for a count of one and return to the starting position. Do 12 to 15 repetitions.

Rear thighs. Leg curls: Lying facedown on a leg curl machine, tuck the backs of your heels underneath the footpads. Curl the weight upward so that your feet move toward your buttocks. Return slowly to the starting position. Do 12 to 15 repetitions.

Ankles. Weighted foot flexes: Start by wrapping wrist or ankle weights around your feet at the base of your toes. Sit on the edge of a high bench or table so that your feet are dangling. Without moving your knees, flex just your toes upward as far as possible so that they point toward your shins. Hold for a second, then point your toes down toward the floor so that you feel a comfortable stretch in front of your ankles. Do 12 to 15 repetitions.

Shoulders. Dumbbell military presses: Sitting on a bench or chair, raise a pair of dumbbells to shoulder height. Press the weights straight overhead until your elbows are almost locked. Return slowly to the starting position. Do 10 to 12 repetitions.

Triceps. Cable pushdowns: While standing, grip the bar attached to a high pulley cable (like the one used for lat pulldowns). With your hands eight inches apart and your elbows tucked against your sides, bring down the bar until it is directly in front of you. (Your forearms should be parallel with the floor.) This is the starting position. Now push down the bar until your arms are extended straight down and the bar is next to your thighs. Return to the starting position following the same path. Do 10 to 12 repetitions.

Biceps. Dumbbell curls: Sitting on the end of an exercise bench, grip a dumbbell in each hand and let your arms hang to your sides. First, curl the weight in your right hand up toward your shoulder. Then lower it and curl up the left. Do 10 to 12 curls with each arm.

Forearms. Barbell wrist curls: While sitting on the end of a bench, grasp the center of a barbell with your hands about eight inches apart, palms up. Lean forward and rest the backs of your forearms on your thighs so that your hands extend past your knees. Moving only your wrists, curl the weight up as far as possible. Lower to the starting posi-

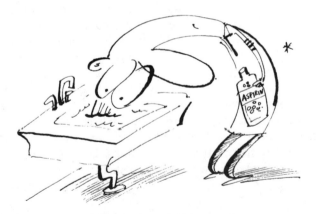

Only Your Lifeguard Knows for Sure

Swimming laps in the pool keeps you in shape all winter, but the chlorine in the water can turn your hair an unpleasant shade of green, particularly if it's blond. You can strip the green tint from swimmer's hair by soaking it in a homemade aspirin rinse: Crush four tablets in several ounces of water, pour the slurry over wet hair, let it sit for five to ten minutes, then rinse. Repeat once a week or as needed.

tion. Do 12 to 15 repetitions. Do a second set with your palms facing down.

Lower back. Dumbbell dead-lifts: Standing with your feet about eight inches apart, place a light dumbbell to the outside of each foot. Keeping your knees as straight as possible and your head up, bend over and grasp the weights with your palms facing in. With your elbows locked, slowly straighten to an upright position. Now bend down, returning the weights to the floor. Do 8 to 12 repetitions. (If you have a bad back, check with your doctor before including this in your routine.)

Stomach. Crunches: Lie on your back with your knees bent, feet flat on the floor. Fold your arms across your chest, tuck your chin, and curl your head up just enough to bring your shoulder blades off the ground. Do not sit all the way up. Hold for a count of two and slowly return to the mat. Do 15 to 20 repetitions.

Lower legs. Toe raises: Holding a dumbbell in your right hand, step up onto a one- to four-inch-high platform so that the balls of your feet are on it and your heels hang free. Tuck the top of your left foot behind the back of your right ankle, and with your left hand resting against a wall for support, rise up on the toes of your right foot. Hold that position for a count of one and return to the starting position. Do 12 to 15 repetitions with each leg.

Cardiovascular system. The best exercises for whipping your heart and lungs into shape are those that also work most of the major muscle groups. Best bets: running, cross-country skiing, swimming and stair climbing.

—Dan Bensimhon

Mountain Biking 101

Are you ready to take your show off the road?
Here's your complete beginner's guide to making
like a mountain goat on wheels.

•••••••••••••••••••

With an involuntary shout, I hurl myself and my 26-pound carbon-fiber machine down the steepest, muddiest trail I can find. My heart is racing. Rocks and stumps seem to fly up at me as my inner radar sends back warnings to veer left or right. Feeling the rear tire lift up, I shift my weight back on the seat a bit to avoid doing a full gainer over the handlebar, duck my head under some branches and white-knuckle it for another 30 seconds until I reach a clearing. Pausing for breath, I can't help thinking that life's good—muddy, but good.

Less than ten years ago, mountain bikes were the sole domain of hippies and bike shop gearheads. But now more than 20 million people own one of these fat-tire wonders, and with good reason. With their upright handlebars and sturdy construction, mountain bikes not only are more comfortable and versatile than ordinary road bikes but also provide a better workout. "When you use a standard road bike, you're basically working only your legs. But off-road mountain biking provides a full-body workout, since you're constantly calling on your upper body to steer around obstacles and pull yourself up hills," says James Hagberg, Ph.D., an exercise physiologist at the University of Maryland who has studied competitive cyclists.

But mountain biking isn't all work and no play. In fact, one of the main reasons fat-tire cycling has become so popular is that it allows riders to be more adventuresome and have a wider variety of riding routes. "When you're mountain biking, you rarely think about how hard you're working because it's more like play than exercise," says Tim Blumenthal, editor of *Mountain Bike* magazine. In addition, many road riders have switched to mountain biking because they find the upright riding position puts less strain on their backs and lets them enjoy cycling more.

Beyond comfort and exercise efficiency, the most attractive feature of a mountain bike is its versatility. By switching from knobby to smooth tires and adding a carrying rack, you can quickly change your mountain bike from a fearless trail vehicle to a sturdy and comfortable commuting bicycle that will take you through potholes and over curbs. Or if you're looking for a bit more speed, switching to lighter rims and skinnier tires can make a mountain bike perform almost like a traditional road bike. "Mountain bikes have lots of uses, whereas road bikes are just . . . well, road bikes," says Blumenthal.

So whether you are a commuter, have an adventurous side or just want to get fit in a hurry, mountain biking is for you. Here's a quick guide to getting started.

● ●

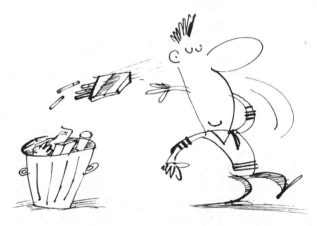

Don't Just Puff— Huff 'n' Puff

If you've quit smoking, you might be worried about putting on a few extra pounds. Well, don't fret about it. Instead, after you eat, use the time you would've spent puffing to take a walk. Scientists took a look at the metabolism of ten male smokers. (They were volunteers generously provided by the U.S. Army.) On different days, the subjects were given a meal and then told to walk for 20 minutes or smoke for 20 minutes. It turned out that the 20-minute walk used up more after-meal calories than the smoking session.

BUYING A BIKE

The first thing you need to do is figure out how much you're willing to spend. For a sturdy mountain bike that'll weather the abuses rugged trails inflict on it, plan on shelling out between $400 and $800. You can spend a lot more if you go for some of the fancy new technology, such as front and rear suspension systems. These can make your ride smoother but aren't worth the extra $300 to $500 unless you're planning to ride on *very* rough terrain. Wherever you plan to ride, steer clear of the department-store $179.95 special. Not only are these bikes less durable than the ones you'll find in bike shops and large sporting goods stores, but bike shop mechanics are much more qualified than stock boys when it comes to bike assembly, frame fitting and service down the road.

Once you buy your bike, you'll need a place to ride. Not all park trails are open to mountain bikers. To locate the ones that are, call your local parks or recreation department. Bike shops and sporting goods stores also offer maps of open trails or bike paths. Rails-to-Trails Conservancy, an organization that specializes in reclaiming abandoned railroad rights-of-way, has compiled a book of more than 4,000 miles of multi-use trails. Write to Rails-to-Trails Conservancy, 1400 16th Street NW, Washington, DC 20036, for ordering information.

When riding a trail, you'll quickly see that this kind of cycling is less about speed than about precision. It requires dexterity and balance—and it takes practice. Which is another way of saying don't expect to come home with clean clothes. What follows are some of the basic skills for off-road mountain biking. As you work on these, the best advice is to be patient, because even though your brain may understand what you need to do, it may take a month or two before your body gets the idea.

CHUGGIN' UPHILL

Shifting. With the right gear choice, even a moderately fit novice mountain biker can make it up some of the steepest hills. Most mountain bikes have 18 or 21 gears controlled by two shifters. Unlike the ones on most street bikes, these

shifters are on the handlebar. That's convenient, since you
don't have to let go of the handlebar to change gears. But
getting comfortable with the shifters takes practice. When
you get to a hill, resist the urge to choose a middle gear and
keep downshifting as the hill gets steeper, since this will
fatigue you quickly. For the best results, shift into an easy
gear at the beginning of the hill and stay with it for the
whole climb.

Body position. To stay on your bike on a steep,
rugged uphill trail, you need to distribute your weight evenly
between the wheels, so the front one doesn't lift and the
back one doesn't lose traction. For beginners, staying seated
and leaning forward is the best way to maintain this balance.
Simply tilt your upper body forward so that your chest is parallel with the ground and your nose is a few inches above the
middle of your handlebar. Dropping your elbows toward the
ground will help. As the hill gets steeper, you may have to
slide forward on your seat a bit to stay balanced. Expert
mountain bikers tackle the steepest hills by standing on the
pedals and leaning forward.

Pedaling. If your front wheel is still coming up or your
rear wheel is spinning out, you may be pedaling too hard.
Smooth, round strokes are much more effective than short,
jerky thrusts in getting you up a hill.

GLIDING DOWNHILL

Shifting. For the most part, the rules of downhill riding
are the opposite of those for uphill. You'll need to be in a
high gear, both to keep enough tension in your chain so that
it doesn't slap your frame and to provide enough resistance
so that you can pedal at the bottom of the hill without spinning your tires.

Finding the line. The best route down is called "the
line." Sometimes the line will be easy to spot—it's that two-
yard gap between the cliff and the boulder. Other times you
have to feel your way through. For example, the instinct is to
ride around puddles, but sometimes that leaves you stuck in
the mud. (The center of the puddle, where ground is too
dense to allow seepage, is often firmer than the surrounding
area.) Momentum is usually the key to getting through rough

terrain, but—do we have to say this?—don't go so fast that
falling is going to make you look like roadkill. In general, focus
on where you want to go and not what you want to steer clear
of. "If you keep saying to yourself 'I have to avoid that rock up
ahead,' nine times out of ten you'll hit it," says Blumenthal.

Body position. As you begin down a hill, your weight
naturally slides forward. If you hit a rock or pothole in this
position, you can count on flying over the handlebar.
Instead, you need to redistribute your weight rearward by
extending your arms and sliding your rear end backward off
the seat. To maintain stability, pinch the back of the saddle
with your thighs and hold your pedals parallel with the
ground to give you maximum clearance over rocks and
uneven terrain.

Braking. Let your back brake do most of the work.
Using the front is fine on smooth terrain, but if your front
wheel hits an obstacle with the front brake applied, you may
lose control. Pump the brakes to keep them from overheat-
ing and losing power on a long descent.

RIDING ON GRASS

Riding on grass is slow and not much fun. But the keys
here are to watch out for hidden ruts and holes and to go
easy on the brakes, or you'll be likely to skid. Never ride off
designated trails.

PUMPIN' IN THE SAND

Loose sand is one of the most difficult surfaces to negotiate. As you come upon a sandy stretch, shift to a higher
gear and grind, don't spin, your way through. Keep pedaling,
since coasting will only make you lose momentum, start to
zigzag and lose your balance. Keep a loose grip on the handlebar, so you can react quickly if your front wheel tries to
wander sideways.

SPLASHING IN THE MUD

Momentum is the key to getting through the mire. As
you approach mud, shift into a slightly lower gear (one or two
clicks down) and slide backward a few inches on your seat to

put more weight on your rear tire and also to keep from flying over the handlebar as the mud slows down your bike. Once you're in the mud, keep pedaling to maintain your momentum and to stabilize your balance. Take a straight line—turning robs you of momentum. For the same reason, avoid braking. (Also, the debris in the mud can rip your brake pads to shreds.) Trails that are extremely muddy should not be ridden until they've had a chance to dry somewhat.

TACKLING DOWNED TREES

Riding over small logs (or "cleaning," as the pros call it) is mostly a matter of quickly shifting your front-to-back balance while maintaining your side-to-side balance. Pedal or coast up to the log so that you're traveling at a moderate speed. Level your pedals and shift your weight backward as your front wheel makes contact. Then as your back wheel makes contact with the log, shift your weight forward to help bring your back wheel over. It's not a bad idea to hone your skills by placing several four- to eight-inch logs about ten feet apart on a level, grassy surface. In full protective gear, practice riding over them. Once you can clean five or six in a row, you're ready to take your show on the trail.

CRUISING OVER DIPS

Dips and ditches come in various shapes and sizes. The bigger ones are better negotiated on foot; smaller ones can be traversed without dismounting. Pick the shallowest line through the dip and ride it as if it were a short downhill followed by a short uphill. Shift your weight backward as you enter the dip and forward as you climb out. You can also cut diagonally across each bank to reduce the steepness, but be careful about hitting your uphill pedal on the way out.

RECOVERING FUMBLES

Fumbling (i.e., losing momentum, stopping, falling) on a long uphill is nearly inevitable, especially if you're on rough terrain. After fumbling, get off your bike and move to a less-steep section of the trail if you can find one. Check to see that your bike is in its easiest gear. If not, lift the rear wheel, shift, and turn the pedals with your hand to get it there. Place your bike at a 45-degree angle to the hill and stand on the uphill side of the bike. Grab your brake levers to lock the wheels in place, then swing your leg over the bike and rest it on the pedal that's pointing downhill. Now lift your uphill foot off the ground, release the brakes, and start to pedal. The trick is not to lunge too hard with the first pedal stroke, since this can cause you to spin out and fumble again.

CRASH COURSE

Falling is part of the mountain-biking experience. A smart rider knows how to protect himself. To do that, you'll need some special equipment.

Helmet. A bike helmet is the most essential piece of cycling equipment when it comes to preventing injury. One study concluded that one life could be saved every day in the U.S. if all cyclists wore helmets. Look for a model that is both Snell- and ANSI-approved for safety. Cost: $40 to $90.

Sunglasses. They keep not only the sun but also low-hanging branches out of your eyes. On overcast days, select clear or amber lenses, which will allow you to see clearly while still providing protection from debris and the sun's ultraviolet rays. Polycarbonate lenses are the lightest and hence the best. Wraparound models keep out wind and UV light most efficiently. Cost: $20 to $90.

Gloves. Padded cycling gloves protect your hands from the scratches and scrapes that can come from riding through the brush. They also help to absorb the shock from a long day of bouncing over rocks and ditches. Cost: $10 to $30.

● ●

Eat and Run

If you're fond of foods such as cheeseburgers and ice cream, you have three health choices: Give them up, get more exercise, or start checking the phone book for the location of the nearest portly man's shop. We know which one *we're* going with.

A 170-pound man who is inactive can eat only 67 grams of fat a day without gaining weight. But a 170-pound man who runs at a moderate pace for 30 minutes each day can add 11 grams of fat to his fat budget, for a total of 78 grams.

Put simply, for every 100 calories you burn during exercise, you can eat about three more grams of fat and not gain weight.

Shoes. Running shoes are too soft. Stiff-soled road-biking shoes are awkward for the part of the time that you're hiking on foot—and trust us, you *will* do some hiking. Look for mountain-biking shoes, which combine a stiffer sole for cycling efficiency with a good tread for hiking. A pair of outdoor cross-trainers is another practical option. Cost: $35 to $120.

Windbreaker. Keeps you warm, dry and windproof. Some versions fold up into a fanny pack for convenience. Cost: $25 to $65.

Bike shorts. Choose cloth, Lycra or Lycra blends, but be sure the shorts have a chamois pad on the inside to provide some shock absorption for your butt. If you choose Lycra shorts, look for those that have at least four panels sewn together. They provide a more contoured fit than shorts with only two panels. Also, if you plan to ride in areas with a lot of brush, wear a pair of light cycling tights to keep your legs from getting scratched. Cost for shorts: $20 to $70; cost for tights: $20 to $50.

Shirt. Tight-fitting polyester bike jerseys are good for staying cool, and they won't snag easily on branches or brush. They're also nice because they have pockets in the back to help you carry your keys or some snacks. Long-sleeved is best to keep you from getting scratched up. Cost: $25 to $75.

—Dan Bensimhon

Part 9

TAKING CARE
OF BUSINESS

The Sound of Success

*To be a success on the job, you've got to
sound like one. Here are the six
secrets of power talking.*

● ● ● ● ● ● ● ● ● ● ● ● ● ● ● ● ● ● ●

IF WE WERE PITCHING a huge order of widgets to our
most frugal client, we'd like George Walther to do the talking for us. He's an expert at influencing people by using simple, direct language. Author of *Power Talking: 50 Ways to
Say What You Mean and Get What You Want,* Walther has
become a specialized kind of English teacher to business-
men, lecturing on the most effective use of our native
tongue to managers at places such as Ford, Du Pont,

General Electric and AT&T. He teaches them how to say what they mean, with punch, and how to make it count. "Achievers speak differently from other people," he points out. "They know how to be positive and forceful without coming across as arrogant."

Walther has distilled the art of verbal success down to a few basics. He says using certain phrases and avoiding others sets the groundwork for effective communication—and success. Six quick English lessons:

1. Instead of "I'll try," say "I will." Words create self-fulfilling prophecies, Walther says. "For example, recently when I had my home remodeled, I noticed that the contractors who said 'I'll try to get back to you by tomorrow' rarely did. Those who said 'I will have an answer for you by 5:00 P.M. tomorrow' followed through. That's because the expectation they set didn't just influence me, it influenced them."

2. Instead of "I have failed," say "I have learned." This focuses you on what you will do differently next time, not on what you should have done. Everyone makes mistakes, points out Walther, but the subtle difference in how you speak about them helps make the experience a positive one.

3. Get rid of the phrase "I disagree." These words are received as a direct challenge and make people want to dig in their heels. Instead of setting up a conflict, aim to win the other guy over. "It shouldn't be just my idea and your idea, and I'm a tough guy, so my idea is going to win," says Walther. "A team player will say 'I understand, and here's another way to look at it.' "

4. Don't start with "It's only my opinion, but . . . " Everyone is uncertain from time to time, but by opening a statement with language like this, you devalue what you're about to say. Worse, you project an image of insecurity. "Just state what you think, plain and simple," says Walther.

5. Avoid the excuse "I just don't have enough time." Plenty of people manage to work hard, excel in their careers, get to the gym and nurture good relationships; they're the ones who don't act as if they have less time than everybody else. "The difference is a matter not just of time management but of attitude management," says Walther.

Successful people realize that there is enough time to do the things that are important, and the difference is reflected in their speech.

6. Nervous? Make it a plus. If you're uneasy before addressing a group, say to yourself "I feel nervous—good." The best public speakers convert that adrenaline rush into positive energy. "To me, public speaking is a kind of thrill, which is the best way to look at it," says Walther. He believes you hurt yourself by putting a negative judgment on nervousness. Look at it as a sign that you're facing a valuable challenge.

—*Richard Laliberte*

True Clout

Men with real power don't need power ties.
Here are 12 secrets a real player should know.

● ● ● ● ● ● ● ● ● ● ● ● ● ● ● ● ● ●

ONE OF THE MOST POWERFUL MEN I've ever known is a guy by the name of Harold W. McGraw, Jr., who, when I met him, was chairman of the board of the company I was working for, McGraw-Hill. There were a number of obvious reasons to feel Harold was a powerful guy. For one thing, his name was on the 50-story behemoth of a building that I worked in. Also, he had all the trappings of authority and status accorded to corporate fat cats. His office on the top floor was very large, ornately paneled with dark wood and, most impressive of all for a workplace in midtown Manhattan, extremely quiet. He had his own elevator to the executive floor and a spare apartment up there somewhere as well.

But these are not the reasons I say he was powerful. After all, when he retired, his successor inherited these trappings, yet never seemed to carry the same weight with people as Harold did. Rather, Harold was powerful because of his style, which was exactly the opposite of what I had expected from an executive of his stature. He was a bit... well...doofy. He had a shuffling gait, and his suits always seemed too big. He could be seen getting off the elevator (not the private one but the one we all used) toting his belongings in a plastic bag rather than in an important-looking attaché case. He also was a master of the personal touch. If you did a favor for Harold, no matter how small, he'd write you a little thank-you in odd but distinctive green ink. The name of every person he met seemed permanently filed in his mental Rolodex. And employees, in response to these endearments, called the boss by his first name.

What these things have to do with power is this: Because he schmoozed with regular people and made them feel important, it was not uncommon to hear employees say things like "I'd do anything for Harold." If that's not power, I'd like to know what is.

In fact, that's exactly what power is, according to experts on personal potency. Power, they say, is really nothing more than the ability to exert influence in order to get what you want. It has almost nothing to do with the things that we usually associate with command and authority. If you want more power in your life, be it at work, at home or anywhere else, the first thing you need to do is forget about whether or not your office is bigger than the next guy's or whether you're wearing this season's power tie and driving the right car. These things can reflect the amount of power you have, but they won't *get* you any.

Likewise, true authority is not about asserting yourself over others or forcing people to do things they'd rather not. Power through domination is inevitably short-lived, since it makes people resentful and resistant and they, in turn, make it more difficult for you to achieve your goals.

WORK WITH PEOPLE

Instead, being influential comes from working *with* people and not against them. "Power is inherently about relationships," says Toni Falbo, Ph.D., a psychologist at the University of Texas at Austin. "It's all about figuring out how people on both sides of an issue can win."

Not to ring the Liberty Bell too loudly, but being American, with all our history of rugged individualism, would seem to allow each of us the opportunity to broker more power. In America, we've taken great pains to see that there are firm limits on the power of government and society at large, preferring instead to stress the importance of individuals, the power of one. Over 200 years after the Declaration of Independence, psychologists are telling us that the Founding Fathers were on to something. Having a sense of individual power, say the experts, really is at the core of our inalienable right to happiness.

For example, research from Harvard University finds that people who are motivated by a drive for power are likeliest to be the most successful. On every rung of the company ladder, workers who have a sense of control over what they contribute to the enterprise tend to be more satisfied with their jobs and more productive. "If you have a sense of power, going to work is a joyful prospect instead of a depressing one," says Peter Wylie, Ph.D., a management consultant in Washington, D.C., and author of *Problem Employees: How to Improve Their Performance.* "You feel your job is exhilarating rather than just an onerous set of tasks."

WEAKNESS MAKES YOU SICK

Lack of power, by contrast, is the most debilitating form of stress. "Most kinds of stress are actually beneficial, and our nervous systems are designed to handle them without any problems," says Oakland, California–based psychologist Robert Bramson, Ph.D., author of *Coping with Difficult Bosses.* "But if you feel frustrated or angry or helpless, it can literally make you sick." Studies suggest that this kind of stress can contribute to heart disease, cancer, depression and lowered immunity.

Few of us need to be sold on the benefits of having more clout. The question now becomes how to get more of what you want from those around you while making them think the world of you at the same time.

For starters, if that last sentence strikes you as a bit manipulative, you're on the right track. The idea *isn't* to trick people into thinking you're on their side so that you can fulfill some hidden agenda. Rather, you need to actually *be* on their side—or win them to yours.

"It's important to respect others and feel that they're worth bargaining with," Dr. Falbo says. "If you respect people, you'll listen to them more. If you don't respect them, they'll sense it and stop talking to you, which is the first way in which you lose power with them."

What's more, keeping an open ear toward others is a surefire way to check Napoleon-like feelings of arrogance and omnipotence. "This is the negative side of power," Dr.

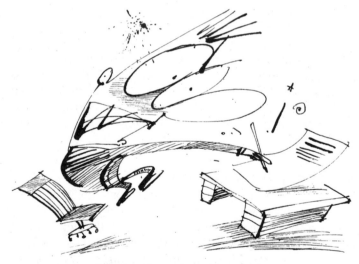

Write Your Own Ticket

If you lose your job, don't worry about it—write about it. A new study finds that people who lose their jobs cope better and find new jobs faster if they put the details of their trauma down on paper. Researchers think writing can help the out-of-work to appraise their emotions, deal with the negative ones and move on.

Bramson says. "When you no longer get honest feedback, you feel unconstrained, you falsely believe that your decisions are right simply because you made them, and you think failures are always somebody else's fault."

We asked the experts for their best advice on matters of power both at work and at home. This is what they had to say.

AT WORK

Here, power issues almost always revolve around bosses. Even if you're jockeying for power with colleagues at your own level, the real issue is usually about your relationship with higher-ups. The supervisor-subordinate dance is also where people feel most helpless when things aren't going smoothly.

There's no sense trying to achieve power parity with a person whose ultimate strength is that he can fire you. You're in a situation in which all the trappings of power go to the other guy from square one. Still, there are tactics for expanding your influence with the boss. Among these:

Resist the urge to brownnose. It's natural to be ingratiating, especially if your boss is an ogre who bullies, steals your ideas or fails to go to bat for his staff. But the indignity of kissing up to the boss bolsters his power, not yours. Instead, you need to work on building mutual respect. "Bullies like people who stand up to them," Dr. Bramson says, "but it's important that you don't gain points over them. You need to behave in a way that's neither provocative nor subservient." One way to do this is to openly stand up for your beliefs when you disagree. Just make sure he knows you're open to his point of view. "Say 'I don't agree with you on that, but tell me more of what you're thinking,' " Dr. Bramson suggests.

See it his way. Shrewd power players know what the boss is after and help him try to get it. If you make your own goals dovetail with his, you'll avoid feeling conflict over the direction of your work. "If you're at odds with what the boss needs, it can make you sullen and resistant or a smartass, all which just get you less of what you want," Dr. Bramson says.

Be direct about your needs. Don't waffle or play

games when asking for something from the boss. "Let's say you want to leave early once a week to take a class," says Bonnie Jacobson, Ph.D., who specializes in issues of power as director of the New York Institute for Psychological Change. "It's a mistake to say something like 'I notice no one is covering the office at 8:30 A.M., so I'd like to come in a half-hour early to do it. And by the way, I'd also like to take a class at night.' That sounds manipulative and insincere. It's better to just say 'I'd like to take this class, but to do it I'll have to leave at 4:30 in the afternoon. I'm prepared to make up the time. Can we work this out?' "

Get smart. Knowledge is power. Granted, that's a cliché, but notice that smart people often have a lot of influence even when they don't have a lot of authority. People listen to them and put stock in what they have to say. To foster an expert image, John Kotter, Ph.D., author of *Power and Influence: Beyond Formal Authority,* suggests an exceedingly simple tactic: Be outspoken when you know a lot about a subject, but keep your mouth shut when you don't. That way, you'll always sound informed, never stupid.

Learn from others. Maybe the veteran colleague in the next office isn't as quick as you and won't go as far, but it's a mistake to write him off. More experienced employees can educate you about the workings of the place and the background of the boss. Defy the dictums of conventional office politics and associate with people whose stars are no longer rising. Understanding the decisions and mistakes they've made can be more valuable than an earful of ambitious chatter from an up-and-comer.

Reverse your tactics. When you're stonewalled, Dr. Bramson advises what he calls a martial arts approach in which you turn obstacles into advantages. If, for example, your boss's micro-management style prevents you from gaining responsibility, understand that he's nervous about mistakes and tap into that with a kind of reverse psychology. "Instead of badgering him, offer to show him drafts of all reports before they go to type," says Dr. Bramson. "If he's afraid of screwups, this signals to him that you're not a danger. After a while, you can suggest taking this detail off his hands, and he'll feel very positive about letting it go."

AT HOME

Nowhere is the importance of good relationships more vital than in the home—in fact, here relationships are the whole point. The greatest motivator, the greatest influencer, the greatest power is love. The challenge is to channel the affection you naturally feel for your partner and children, so they do what you consider best for themselves or the family as a whole. Here's what to do.

Strive for balance. This isn't a matter of everyone having equal power over everything. It's typical that each partner is dominant in particular areas of the household, says

● ●

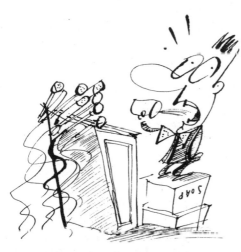

Beverage Do's and Don'ts for Speakers

Room-temperature water with a touch of lemon is the best beverage for a nervous speaker with a dry throat, say Marjorie Brody and Shawn Kent, coauthors of the new book *Power Presentations.* Avoid ice water, which will constrict your throat. Cool water will help your voice sound rich, and the lemon will clear any mucus buildup. You might want to bring a small container of water in your briefcase. The pitcher next to the podium is usually filled with ice.

Here are other drinks to avoid before a presentation.

■ Milk. It will coat your throat and cause phlegm. Avoid eating ice cream and yogurt as well.

■ Soda. Its carbonation will make you belch.

■ Coffee and tea. The caffeine will make you jumpy.

■ Alcohol. It will relax you when you want to be sharp.

No water available? As a last resort, bite your tongue. Your glands will produce saliva, which will moisten your mouth.

Martin Goldberg, M.D., director of the Marriage Council of Philadelphia. The important thing is that both people feel that the balance is equitable and comfortable. If your partner thinks something is skewed—she feels you have too much control over the checkbook, for example—it's in your best interest to even things up.

Build trust. "Intimacy can occur only when a person feels safe," Dr. Jacobson says. You probably already said everything that needed saying on this score when you were at the altar: that you'll always be there, that you won't fool around, that you'll love and respect her. Still, some of this bears repeating every now and again. "Saying 'I want you to understand how much I respect you' would be an excellent statement to make at any time," Dr. Falbo says.

Ask her opinion. About you, that is. "It's not so much asking for a judgment of what kind of man you are. Rather, it's how your behavior is affecting her," Dr. Jacobson says. She and other experts assert that seeking comments from others about your own behavior is one of the most powerful ways to build relationships and increase intimacy. "It makes you smarter about yourself and makes others more comfortable with you," she says.

Invest time in children. There's no better way to score points with them, to gain their respect, to understand what's going on with them, to know what their friends are like or to guide their decisions than just being around them. Don't worry if the moments you spend with them are "quality time" or not. In fact, managing family time wisely also means respectfully leaving well enough alone when the kids would just as soon you get lost.

Let kids decide for themselves. "The more that people feel their own power, the more likely they'll do what's right for themselves," Dr. Bramson says. It's your job to point out the possible consequences of kids' actions, not to take on responsibilities that belong to them.

"If they're not doing their homework, badgering them only makes it worse, because any self-respecting kid will resist you," Dr. Bramson says. "Instead, say 'Here's the problem you'll face if you don't do it,' then leave it alone. The basic rule is to show respect and love, which is easier to do if you recognize that it's their life, not yours."

Be persistent—and patient. The more you ask for, the more you're likely to get. "That's not an endorsement of being obnoxious," Dr. Goldberg says. "But if you know what you want, ask for it and are willing to wait a day, a week, a year to get it, time will take care of a lot of your needs."

The same could be said of all power-building relationships. "When people are at their best, each person helps the other become more powerful," Dr. Goldberg concludes. "One of the best things you can do in life is to help others develop their potential. If you're able to do it, both you and they feel tremendously gratified and more closely united."

—Richard Laliberte

Creativity Unlimited

Think you're not all that creative? Think again.
We all harbor great ideas, say the experts.
Here's how to get them out in the open.

• • • • • • • • • • • • • • • • • •

WHEN THE LEGENDARY RICHARD WAGNER was composing his opera *Parsifal,* he found creative inspiration through day-long soaks in a lavender-scented bath. On the other hand, when Seymour Cray, the reclusive genius who gave the world its first super computer, found himself stymied by an operating problem, he'd dig a hole. Well, not exactly a hole; more like a man-size tunnel, which ran from the back of the house to the woods at the edge of his property.

People come by their moments of creativity in many different ways. Some seem to have generators in their heads that serve up freshly baked ideas 24 hours a day, much like a cerebral Dunkin' Donuts. Others need just the right lighting, some baroque background music and a half-hour of biofeedback to get their creative powers juiced.

And then there are the majority of people. You and I. The ones who sit in front of a blank piece of paper for hours, straining away in a manner more suggestive of childbirth than of brainstorming.

While we don't need to be true creative geniuses to get ahead, a few good ideas now and then can turn the corporate ladder into an escalator. Now and then, however, is not the problem. Given 20 or 30 years, we all manage to trip over a good idea or two. The problem is when you need a good idea by tomorrow and the clock on the wall says 4:30 P.M.: 4:30, and there's no one in sight; 4:30, and no chance of throwing together a spur-of-the-moment brainstorming session. You feel a cold sweat coming on as you realize that tonight you'll be brainstorming by yourself—trying to draw water from a well as dry as your mouth will be tomorrow when you face your boss empty-handed.

What do you do? How can you turn that drop of an idea into a thunderstorm? How do you change a sputtering candle into a chandelier of inspiration?

STEP ONE: UPLOAD AND INCUBATE

Don't get nervous. This first step will not require you to sit buck naked in a darkened room and listen to the sounds of mating humpback whales. While we all harbor suspicious, archetypal perceptions of the creative process as a somewhat eccentric and bohemian experience, there are ways to strike inspirational gold that don't require you to first draw the curtains and dim the lights.

To get things rolling, simply take an hour to look over all the information you have that directly pertains to the problem. Say you need to have five children's toy concepts for the big meeting tomorrow. Look over recent market surveys to see which toys are currently doing big business and which are collecting dust. Peruse reports on new toy concepts your company is already considering for launch. Examine any budgetary information that may have some bearing on new product development, and finish up with a glance at the most recent focus-group results.

While you're reviewing this information, don't bother to dwell on any particular aspect. Think of your brain as a computer: You are simply feeding it data for storage, data that will be processed at a later point.

Idea Power

At the end of an hour, once you've finished uploading the information, put the notebooks, memos, research and other assorted papers away. You've just initiated a powerful creative process known as incubation.

If you've ever worked on a problem that drove you into an impotent frenzy on Monday only to find that come Wednesday, the problem seemed to solve itself, you've experienced the results of incubation. "There are creativity specialists who believe that when you take a break from something you're working on, your mind continues to consider the problem—even when you've gone on to a totally different task," says Eugene Raudsepp, president of Princeton Creative Research. "It's a subconscious process that we aren't even aware is happening. All we know is that one day we have an unsolvable problem that keeps getting worse, and the next day it's solved.

"To get started," says Raudsepp, "all you need to do is assemble the information that pertains to the problem and give it the once-over. This is how you prime the pump, so to speak. Then put it away and go do something entirely different. Something that has nothing to do with the problem."

At this point, you've planted the seeds of information. From now until you finally sit down for the actual brainstorming session, your subconscious mind will be working on the problem.

It's 5:30 P.M. On to step two.

• •

Needle Yourself
to Success

If you're looking for that extra-sharp competitive edge, consider a visit to an acupuncturist. Researchers at the University of Vienna Department of Sport and Performance Medicine say men who were treated with acupuncture once a week for five weeks performed 7 percent better on a test of stationary-cycling prowess than a similar group that didn't get needled.

STEP TWO: TAKE THE LONG WAY HOME

Colt invented the revolver after watching the paddle wheel on a riverboat. The concept behind the hot air balloon was born one afternoon when the Montgolfier brothers watched scraps of burnt paper rise from the fireplace and sail up the chimney on a current of heated air. The man who invented Velcro was inspired by the common burr.

As these people discovered, the makings of a great idea are all around you. Virtually any object has the potential to reach out and trigger your mind. Roger Van Oech, internationally recognized creativity consultant, likes to ask his seminar participants this question: "Have you walked through a junkyard lately?" What he's proposing is that we take time to do something out of the ordinary, to look for and at things normally not seen.

At the Center for Creative Leadership, associate program director Jim Shields often suggests that people try brainstorming in places other than the office. "I've found that many times the different surroundings and new stimuli encourage people to make totally new creative connections," he says.

But we are a species that likes routine. We take the same route to work each morning, eat the same foods in the same restaurants at lunch, keep the same pictures on our office walls for years and then drive home at 5:00 P.M. the same way we came. While this makes for a work routine that's as comfy and familiar as a pair of slippers, it unfortunately does not allow the brain to come in contact with the new stimuli it occasionally needs to form new ideas.

Check Your Mental Balance

What you've got to do is start thinking of your mind as a checking account. Coming up with ideas is the equivalent of writing checks against your mental account. But as we all know, you can't draw on an account unless you occasionally make deposits. When you expose your mind to new stimuli, you are in effect making a deposit—putting a little something into the "image" account that may later yield an idea.

So today, before we try to make a withdrawal, we're

going to make a deposit on the way home from work. Grab a
tape recorder and head out to the car. Once you get out of
the parking lot, make a left instead of that right you've made
a thousand times before. Forget about the route you normally take, the one where you know the timing of every traffic light along the way.

Today, we're going for a scenic cruise. We're going to
get a little lost. We're going to take some time to look around.
And if you see anything that captures your imagination, make
a note of it on tape. Describe it and then move on. Otherwise,
don't worry about solving problems or how much time you
seem to be wasting on a joyride. Remember, your subconscious is already incubating away. Meanwhile, did you happen to notice that combination croissant shop and wholesale
meat outlet on the left? What about that roadside attraction
up there on the right? The one boasting "World's Largest
Collection of Naturally Occurring Lubricants!!!"? Believe it or
not, this is the sweet stuff from which ideas are born.

Your drive should take about an hour and leave you in
front of your house at 6:30 P.M., with a full checking account
in your head.

STEP THREE: LAUGH

Once you've gotten home, it's time for a mood adjust-
ment. You've had a mother of a day, topped off by a homework assignment that'll keep you from watching the playoffs
tonight. If you think that wallowing in a pool of resentment is
any kind of prelude to brainstorming, you're dead wrong.

"I've found that the most productive brainstorming
meetings are the ones where everyone is laughing and having a good time," says Roger L. Firestien, acting director of the
Center for Studies in Creativity at Buffalo State College. "As a
matter of fact, the more I've watched the connection between
humor and increased creativity, the more I've realized that
there is very little difference between 'Aha!' and 'Ha ha!' "

A number of studies support Firestien's observations. In
one experiment performed by Alice M. Isen, Ph.D., former
professor of psychology at Cornell University's Johnson
School of Management, two groups of people were given a

candle, a book of matches, a box of tacks and a corkboard attached to the wall. Both groups were asked to arrange the materials in a manner that would allow the candle to burn without dripping wax onto the floor.

One group was shown a funny movie beforehand. The other went to work with nary a chuckle. When the experiment was completed, more people from the movie group were successful in coming up with a creative solution that fit the bill. (If you're wondering how it's done: Empty the box of tacks, tack the box to the board, set the candle on top of the box, and then light it.)

Psychologists say that a positive affect seems to boost our ability to relate and integrate divergent material. All we need to know from this is that a good laugh can be the prelude to a good idea. "If you're going to be doing a little creative problem solving," says Firestien, "I think it would be totally appropriate to begin by watching a Monty Python video or some other piece of comedy that tickles your funny bone."

So step three is to take a half-hour and watch something funny. Reading is also permissible. You probably never dreamed you'd hear this, but a judicious half-hour spent with a copy of *National Lampoon* may end up making you the company wunderkind!

STEP FOUR: SET THE PARAMETERS

It's now 7:00 P.M. and time to get down to business. "The first thing to do is situate yourself by a window," says Firestien. "Once again, you want to present your mind with as much stimuli as possible. It could be that you need to find a way to increase sales by 5 percent. As you look out the window, you might see a tree bending and swaying in the wind. The flexibility of the tree just might get you thinking about creating a more 'flexible' payment plan for clients. Perhaps the plan might attract the new customers you need."

Having gotten your window seat, settle down and take a good look at the problem you need to solve. Maybe you need to suggest ways to broaden your company's line of products. Perhaps you're charged with increasing the effectiveness of plant operations by finding a way to use equipment that is currently dormant for 8 out of 24 hours. Whatever the challenge, write it down.

Next, write down ten things you can't do to solve the problem. Let's say your company manufactures toys and you need to come up with five product suggestions; write down "heavy construction equipment" as one of them. "What's the point?" you ask. Here's a riddle to help you answer that question: Using two American coins (currently in circulation), one of which cannot be a quarter, can you make the total equal 35 cents? Well? Give up? The answer is a quarter and a dime. Cheating? Not at all. The question stated that one of the coins cannot be a quarter. Well, one of them isn't a quarter—it's a dime.

Unspoken Rules

The problem is that we're all born assumption makers and lifelong boundary builders. We take unspoken rules for granted without realizing that we're acknowledging these rules. How often do you say "We can't do that because it's just not done"? What you have to remember is that the birth pains of every new and successful idea are largely the result of shattering a former rule. The most creative ideas always break with tradition.

"Finding a creative answer to a problem frequently involves finding a creative problem definition," says Shields. "In our classes, we encourage people to really notice how they see a problem and then challenge them to come up with a long list of different ways to think about it."

A problem frequently used as an example at the Center for Creative Leadership comes from the tea industry in Great Britain: In 8 hours, a company can produce all the tea bags it needs. Although the machines have a spare production capability, they are idle 16 hours a day. What can be done?

"The first and most common way people look at the problem is to think of what other drinks can be put into tea bags," says Shields. "Answers usually include things such as coffee and hot chocolate." But as Shields quickly points out, why assume that you have to make tea bags? "If you free yourself from that unspoken rule, then suddenly you've opened up a whole new realm. You could take the extra bagging material the machines can produce, dye it and make curtains or disposable clothes. Maybe it could be used as mosquito netting or cut into sheets and used as eyeglass-cleaning tissue."

So try breaking the rules. Maybe suggesting the production of heavy construction equipment to a toy company is a little outlandish . . . but maybe not. You can always take these outlaw ideas and modify them. For example, why not build child-size, battery-powered dump trucks that kids could actually drive around the backyard?

Try for 40

Having familiarized yourself with the parameters you intend to break, you must also set a quota of ideas to develop. "You should try for at least 40, for a number of reasons," says Firestien. "Number one is that most of us are our own worst critic. We deep-six ideas even before we've given ourselves the chance to fully develop them. By forcing yourself to come up with 40, you've almost got to put your internal critic on hold and write down every idea that comes along. Don't worry if some of them are weak. You can fine-tune them later."

Another reason to shoot for 40 lies in the very nature of the creative process. "Typically, the first third of your ideas can be classified as the 'same-old same-old,' " says Firestien. "These are the ideas that have sort of been rattling around in your mind for months. The second third tends to get more interesting. But it's the last third of your ideas that will really show insight, creativity and complexity. These are the ones you're shooting for." Think of it this way: Any time you take a trip to some new destination, part of the journey passes over familiar ground. You've got to travel through your town before you get out of town, down the road and out of state.

Finally, going for 40 may help get you on an idea roll. "I've found that when the best ideas start coming, they come fast and furious," says Firestien. "By going for 40, you're giving yourself a chance to hit your stride and develop a flow. Most of the time you'll find that as you approach 40, the flow will sweep you up to and past your goal."

STEP FIVE: BLAST OFF!

You've primed yourself subconsciously, visually and emotionally. You've gotten yourself hip to the tired old assumptions that shackle the creativity of every other poor slob you work with, and you've set your marching orders. At this point, if you listen carefully, you can actually hear your brain whir and buzz. Now it's time to "get down with you bad self," as James Brown so aptly put it.

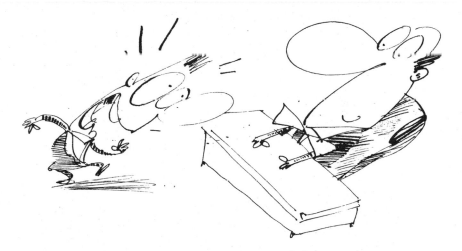

Smile Your Way to the Top

If you are trying to impress a new boss—and someday join his golf foursome—you'd do well to attack your duties with a smile rather than a smirk. In fact, having a positive attitude may be just as important as being talented when it comes to winning the favor of a supervisor, according to psychologist David V. Day, Ph.D., of Pennsylvania State University. "You could be the office superstar, but if you're a frowner, it's unlikely you'll ever join the boss's inner circle," Dr. Day says. In a study of the early relationships between supervisors and subordinates, Dr. Day found that those who lead are quicker to pick up underlings' negative vibes than to notice positive ones. That may be because our instinct to survive makes us more attuned to threatening emotions. Whatever the reason, Dr. Day says those first negative impressions are often long lasting.

First, start writing down the first ideas that come to your mind. These will be the ones that have been brewing for the last couple of hours.

If you run out of ideas quickly, don't sweat it. There are plenty of other ways to coax a concept out of hiding. Turn to the tape you made in the car and give it a listen. On a separate piece of paper, jot down anything striking that you remember from your little excursion. Now study each notation and see if you can't make a connection, no matter how ridiculous, to the problem at hand. For example, suppose the problem is finding a way to unload huge amounts of toys that have gone out of vogue. As you listen to the tape, maybe you'll be reminded of a factory outlet selling women's clothing. What about a chain of toy outlets?

Once you've exhausted the tape, turn to the dictionary or telephone book. "I've found that a good way to stimulate random connections is to close my eyes, let the Yellow Pages fall open where they may and point to a listing," says Firestien. "If it happens to be 'Plumbing,' then start thinking about plumbing and how a plumber connects pipes or fixes leaks, and see if a germ of an idea comes to you."

Oftentimes, one word can get you going. During a brainstorming session at the Campbell Soup Company, someone opened the dictionary to the word "handle." Someone else free-associated the word "utensil." This led to "fork," and one guy joked about a soup you could eat with a fork. Well, they reasoned, you can't eat soup with a fork unless it's chock-full of chunks of meat and vegetables and . . . Bingo! What about Chunky Soups? Campbell's line of Chunky Soups has since enjoyed enormous success in the marketplace—and the idea started with the dictionary entry "handle."

Take a Mental Trip

You can also use what's called the excursion technique. Look at a travel magazine and pick an exotic destination. Create a story having to do with the setting, or at the very least imagine yourself taking a walk around this location. Imagine the kinds of things you'd see there and write them down. A group at the Department of Defense once took an "excursion" to the desert, and in the process, one of the participants "saw" a sidewinder. Someone else commented that the sidewinder locates its prey by sensing body heat and . . . Wait a minute! What about creating an air-to-air missile that homes in on enemy jets by detecting the planes' heat emissions? Naturally, they called it the Sidewinder missile.

Or try imagining yourself as someone else. Someone famous. At a recent brainstorming session for magazine editors, Van Oech asked one group to imagine that they were Madonna. What ideas might they have for the knitting magazine they ran? One suggestion was to run an article called "Knit a Naughty Nightie." While that idea wasn't quite right for the magazine, it did lead to others that were. So try approaching your problem as Napoleon or Mick Jagger and see what happens.

Analogies can also shed some light on a solution. What else is the problem like? For example, when the Israeli air force needed a way to speed up the healing process for wounds, an analogy was drawn between a wound and a severed electrical cord. To restore the flow of current, the wire had to be spliced back together. According to Bryan Mattimore of Mattimore Communications, who tells the story, the solution took the form of a revolutionary bandage containing magnesium, an element known to conduct electricity. The increased flow of electrical current through the body helped speed up the healing process.

Having run the gamut of techniques, all that's left now are two warnings. Warning #1: As hard as this may be to believe, the first few times you try this process you may not come up with a $10 million idea that will change the face of the business world. It's okay. Creativity, much like anything else, takes practice. Soon enough, you'll be awed by your own brilliance. When that happens, keep in mind Warning #2: Try not to look too pleased with yourself. Nothing is more annoying than someone who shows up at every meeting with 40 great ideas.

—Mark Golin

Promote Yourself

Ready to move up the ladder? Before you go see your boss, take a look at the Ultimate Promotion Strategy.

• • • • • • • • • • • • • • • • • • •

MOST PROMOTIONS JUST COME. Like rainfall. Well, okay, maybe like rainfall in the desert. A bit irregularly, perhaps, but during the early stages of your career, chances are one shows up every couple of years.

But sometimes they don't.

You're doing a good job. A very good job. You're ready, willing and able—but the boss, well, he seems to be walking around with his eyes closed.

Or is he?

Most bosses aren't blind, even though they may act that way. Their vision problems are with their imaginations, not their eyes.

What they see is what you are—not what you could be.

And when it comes to big promotions—the ones that give you quantum levels of new responsibility—that gap stops many bosses cold.

Giving a major promotion is an act of faith, actually. "Sure, he does his job well," your boss says to himself. "But how do I know he's got the leadership flair to head up a 12-person R & D department?" Or "What kind of proof do I have that he can handle sensitive negotiations with vendors when he's always been an inside man?" Or "How can I possibly know if he'll cave in under the high stress of reorganizing our screwed-up accounting department when all he's ever done is his own job?"

Fearing a big mistake exactly as much as you want the big promotion, your boss may decide to play it safe. He has two ways to do that. The first is to do nothing. Though a position of high responsibility could be created for you, it never happens. Status quo rules the scene. The second way is to hire someone from outside who has specific experience handling the job you thought had your name on it.

ACT AS IF

So just when you need an act of faith, your boss decides that—as far as your future is concerned—he's strictly an agnostic. The challenge is to bridge that gap of faith. The best way I know to do that—which is why I call it the Ultimate Promotion Strategy—is simple in concept. To get the job you want, act as if you already have it.

Now you won't read that advice in any corporate manual. And few bosses will suggest it. For one thing, logic tells us that if everyone acted as if he had a higher-level job, the result would be chaos. Logic also suggests that telling people who are being paid to do job A that they ought to do job B, C or D seems unfair and, in some instances, even illegal.

But logic lies. The result won't be chaos, because you'll still be doing the job you were hired to do—only more. And though this strategy may seem unfair, it isn't when you put the burden on yourself.

The key to this strategy is that the only way your boss can feel confident you can handle entirely new responsibilities is if he sees you are already doing exactly that.

Of course, there are bosses who, regarding potential, can read between the lines and won't require extraordinary initiatives before handing you a major promotion.

I am not one of them.

After promoting several hundred people over several decades, including 25 to 30 major promotions, I feel more than ever that I need "proof" before the big decisions.

When I was the novice editor of a newspaper in Philadelphia, I had an employee who was a superb copy editor. She could make any reporter's story clear and literate and do it fast. After a few months, I rewarded her by promoting her to reporter, with a 20 percent raise. Two weeks later she was literally a nervous wreck, crying, gobbling pills and missing half her deadlines. What we both discovered was that she had no stomach at all for reporting hard news. Interviewing homicide detectives, families of murder victims, sleazy politicians and assorted militants, she learned, was vastly different from sitting in front of a typewriter.

Some years later, I made the same mistake at a magazine. I hired a journalism professor from a major university because I assumed he'd be a good journalist. In fact, he was terrible. Maybe he was a good teacher, but as a writer he flunked out. I finally fired him, and he went back to teaching. We were both much happier, I'm sure.

So yes, I'm an agnostic until you can show me you can do exactly what that different job entails. You don't have to do it perfectly or even expertly. There's time to grow once you're in the job. But at least show me you can do it.

GETTING YOUR MESSAGE ACROSS

The first step is critical. Ask yourself "Just what does this hoped-for new position entail?" I mean, in every way.

Let's say you're a sales manager and you want to be promoted to sales director. Do you know what a sales director is expected to do and achieve in your company? If your answer is "direct the sales staff," you actually don't know anything. You need specifics. Without specific knowledge, you're shooting at a target you can't even see.

There are three ways to gain this critical information. One is by intelligent osmosis. You simply see, hear—maybe overhear—and sniff out what's expected.

The second way is to ask the sales director what he does and what he's expected to achieve. Even if he's the person you report to, he will probably tell you—in all the detail you desire. People are eager to let others know all the responsibilities they have.

The third way is to ask someone a bit higher on the management totem pole. You may need to do that if your own boss gets uptight about such questions. Maybe he fears you're angling for his job. Or maybe he's not anxious to lose you to another area.

When you have this information, spend an evening jotting down what you'd be doing if you had that director's job right now.

Would you spend a lot more time thinking of new sales strategies instead of just selling?

Would you spend a lot more time looking at market research? Analyzing sales statistics?

Would you be more attentive to details? Would you have all sorts of information at your fingertips? Read more trade publications? Do more networking?

Would you spend more time training people and motivating them?

Would you dress differently? Speak differently? Act differently?

There is no substitute for actually putting these things down on paper and studying them.

DO YOU REALLY WANT IT?

You may discover, for instance, that you don't really want that particular job. It may entail spending large amounts of time and energy doing things you have no stomach for—extensive travel, for instance, lots of presentations, numerous reports that need to be produced but are seldom read.

If you aren't scared off, keep studying your notes. What you're looking for are things you can begin doing immediately, without disrupting either the substance or appearance of your current position.

Here's a perfect example I saw at one of my first jobs, at a computer company. I'd been there only a month or two when a coworker who'd been working there for a year radically streamlined a spiderweb of paperwork that engulfed several departments of the company. Dick hadn't been asked to do this; it was strictly his own idea. He did the work on his lunch hours and on weekends over a period of about ten weeks, finally presenting management with an outline of who really needed to approve what, and he created actual forms that could be used in transmitting reports, requests, bills and similar documents. Paperwork would be reduced by more than 50 percent.

His plan was quickly instituted, and the rest of us all wondered why we hadn't done the same. The truth was that we assumed there was some profound reason behind the labyrinth of forms and concluded it was a part of corporate culture.

Dick, incidentally, was promoted to assistant marketing manager in a different department some four months later.

Ironically, he had no marketing experience whatsoever, but the manager hated paperwork with a passion and thought Dick's action initiative was a clear sign of a young man with a big future.

It was only just before I left the company for another job that I discovered the real reason for all the paperwork we'd had to contend with. Four or five years earlier, not one but

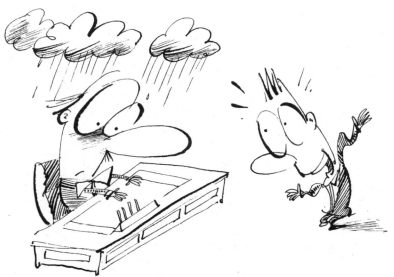

Time Is of the Essence

When's the best time to ask for a raise?

That depends upon the strength of your argument and your boss's mood, says Herbert Bless, a research associate at the University of Mannheim in Germany.

In studies exploring the effect of mood on information processing, Bless found that people tend to evaluate information more thoroughly when they're mildly depressed than when they're euphoric.

So if you think you've got a good case, approach your boss when he's feeling a little down. He'll probably consider your request in the kind of detail that would end up bene-fiting you. If your argument is weak, wait until he's in a great mood. He just may be distracted enough to miss any holes in your logic.

two quite corrupt individuals were caught stealing equipment, signing phony vouchers and generally robbing the company blind, apparently to pay gambling debts. After firing the thieves, high-level management dropped that net of triple-checks over all manner of activity to ensure nothing like that could ever happen again.

But there were no more thieves at the company, and the procedures were nothing more than institutionalized waste. The rules, in effect, began robbing the company of resources where the thieves left off.

Situations like that, involving procedures that are clearly outmoded but never changed, are common in organizations. For the future or current executive, they are a perfect target for initiatives that demonstrate your smarts.

BE SPECIFIC

Dick did another thing that I've learned over the years is very intelligent, and the principle may be stated as follows: It is essential to make your suggested changes and plans as specific as possible.

Making general suggestions is completely useless strategy. Your boss has probably thought of these things himself a million times. But he lacks the time, energy or vision to act on them, and you're not helping him a bit.

So work with your ideas for a while. Make them as specific as they'd be if you were the boss and were going to implement them next week. Don't worry for a minute that your idea may be too specific. The boss can always change the details—you can bet on that. But without them, your idea may not seem "real."

And don't worry, either, about your boss saying "Why didn't you ask me about this before you went ahead and did it?" Your answer is: "This is only an idea. But I had to write it out to see if it would really work and to let you know what I had in mind."

Less than a year ago, a writer at Rodale Press gave me a proposal for a new magazine—on ballroom dancing. There were four pages of details, with all sorts of article ideas. I didn't think we were ready to do a whole major magazine, but I countersuggested a bimonthly column in *Prevention,* Rodale's health and fitness magazine. We also decided to advance a little on the learning curve by offering Rodale employees ballroom dance classes and arranging for dance classes followed by a Big Band Bash at *Prevention's* annual Health and Fitness Festival.

The point is, none of this would have been implemented if Maggie hadn't presented all her specifics about why ballroom dancing is such a great, fun way to exercise. And it was not just the details but also her enthusiasm in presenting the whole picture that gave me the confidence to act on her suggestion.

You can do the same thing with ideas for sales strategies, new products, cost cutting, reorganization, advertising campaigns, you name it. But when you name it, do it with gusto. An idea that carries the double wallop of specificity and enthusiasm has a much greater chance of penetrating the corporate brain trust than a vague and emotionally neutral one.

MORE BANG FOR YOUR BUCK

Speaking of full-metal jacket intellectual bullets, you can triple the impact of your idea by taking a little longer to work it out.

Instead of suggesting only a one-step idea, make it a two-, three- or four-step number. If your idea saves time, suggest how that newfound resource should be spent. If money is saved, suggest how at least some of it could be redirected. But make certain this newfound energy is directed at something new and of clear strategic importance rather than at more of the same-old same-old.

A cousin of mine worked at a country products mail-order business, a mom-and-pop operation that did well but not great and was always waist-deep in cash flow problems. He suggested cutting back on the size and paper quality of their catalogs, which would save $60,000 a year. He further suggested informing their customers that this move was to help preserve the environment and to keep prices down and that Mom and Pop hoped their customers would support them in this decision. But he also suggested using half the money saved to retain a direct-sales marketing consultant and the other half for a financial consultant. Mom and Pop promoted him to general manager.

The reason this combination approach triples the impact of your suggestions is simple. Executives excel not by doing A, then B, then C but by creating integrated structures and systems to achieve key goals. By showing you understand how all the parts can be readjusted to create this more effective engine, you're demonstrating to your boss— and maybe to your boss's boss—that you think like a true executive, a leader, not just someone who happened to have one nifty but isolated idea.

LOOKING THE PART

Across America, in every organization except the military and the police, there are millions of men who go to work each day dressed like they're attending an 8:00 A.M. college lecture on Chaucer and diphtheria. If you are under 30 and dress very casually, you will look like a kid. Over 30, like the manager of a live bait shop. Either way, it doesn't exactly add up to executive élan.

Many of these people are thinking "When I get promoted, I'll dress better. But right now, (a) I don't need to, (b) I can't afford to, or (c) I'll look overdressed." All those reasons are valid—in your head. But in the real world, style talks, validity walks.

Look at it from your boss's point of view. Why make it even harder for him to envision you in a seriously better job? Now some bosses in some kinds of companies don't care a lick how you dress. Personally, I tend to be very tolerant of offbeat and even wacky attire—perhaps because creativity is so important in the communications business. But I have to confess that people who always wear dreary or old-fashioned clothing give me the impression that they're not exactly bred for a leadership role.

If your boss always dresses casually, there is no special need for you to dress any better. But if he wears a stylish jacket and tie to work and you look like Mark Trail, you can bet there's at least a subconscious perception on his part that you may not really want a promotion, that you might be uncomfortable with the responsibility of command.

Is that selling out? Hypocrisy? Yes. I mean, no. I mean, not really. If you violate your values and your beliefs to get ahead, that's hypocrisy. But unless you deeply believe that everyone should dress like Mark Trail, wearing clothes that evince your aspirations is just good psychology.

Dressing and generally behaving like a person of some substance has another very important advantage.

When a boss is deciding whether or not to promote someone to an important job, he actually thinks in two directions. Chiefly, he thinks about you, the candidate, and tries to imagine you in the new position. But he probably is also thinking about what his boss—and his peers—will think of his decision.

What he certainly doesn't want is for the big boys to say "You promoted Benson to head of corporate communications? Hmm...that's an interesting move. Do you think he has what it takes?" Because that makes him look like a poor judge of character—and maybe not such a great exec.

These other people probably barely know you—their whole perception of you is based on seeing you in the hall and other chance encounters. Still, they do have a perception. And your boss can probably guess what it is.

To the extent, then, that you dress in uncool styles and commit other behavioral faux pas, such as avoiding eye contact with higher-ups, telling loud jokes in the lunchroom about boils and midgets and sporting a bumper sticker that says "I Brake for Hallucinations," you're making it hard for your boss to promote you even if he doesn't care about such things.

NOW THAT THE IRON IS HOT . . .

So far, our approach to significant promotions is a true strategy. The rest is half tactics, half happenstance.

Only you know when you've proven your point. Only you can sense if and when you should specifically ask for a promotion, not to mention whom. And if you choose not to, only you can sense the point at which your initiatives and perseverance have turned from a path into a treadmill.

If you sense the latter, you absolutely must talk to your boss to get his assessment of your position, if you haven't already. Though you may feel you're on a treadmill after two years of doing everything right, you don't want to hop off just when the boss is confident he'll finally get budget approval to promote you to associate manager of R & D. On the other hand, if he's negative about your near-term prospects, you might as well ask him on the spot if he would help you advance your career elsewhere in the company—or even outside. Any decent boss will find it hard to refuse such a request.

But I'll tell you something else. When you ask him that question point-blank and he instantly imagines you gone, and you're being so respectful by asking his guidance and blessing (and not issuing an ultimatum), he just may decide that perhaps he was being a bit too negative a moment before. If that occurs, immediately pin him down. If the time frame for promotion exceeds six months or depends on some unlikely event such as a much bigger budget, he's just blowing smoke. Repeat your request for his help, and get on with your career.

What I like most about this strategy is that whatever else it accomplishes, it forces you to confront the kind of behavior that's needed for the position you're shooting for and to try it on for size. And assuming the fit is comfortable, it then encourages you to quit waiting and begin bringing out the best you have within you right now.

—Mark Bricklin

Part 10

ASK

MEN'S HEALTH

The 20 Questions Modern Men Ask Most

Allergic to condoms? Better find out!
This and 19 other pressing questions
you might be wondering about.

• • • • • • • • • • • • • • • • • • •

As EDITOR OF *MEN'S HEALTH* MAGAZINE, I get hundreds of letters from men all over the country. These 20 are representative of the kinds of things on most men's minds. Maybe on yours, too?

—*Mike Lafavore*

POURING BEER

Q. I've noticed that bartenders always pour beer down the side of the glass to keep the foam down. But I've heard that it's better to pour the beer into the center of the glass because this helps to unlock the flavor. Is there any merit to this theory?

—*C.J., Tallahassee, Florida*

A. There is. By pouring beer into the center of the glass, you get more bubbles, which release the aroma of the beer and enhance its taste, according to Charlie Papazian, president of the American Homebrewers Association. On the other hand, you don't want to put too much of a head on your beer. Optimum pouring is a matter of balance, says Papazian. He suggests you begin by letting the beer flow down the side of the glass, then move the stream into the center in order to top off the beer with a half-inch head.

LIP SERVICE

Q. Please give me the definitive answer on how to trim a mustache. I'm frustrated by the hairs that are too long to lay down nicely but not long enough to conform to the curve of my lip, so consequently, they wind up sticking straight out. In frustration, I usually wind up yanking them out. Isn't there a less painful way?

—*J.T., Boise, Idaho*

A. The best lip service is to groom your mustache from the bottom up. Start trimming at the line where your mustache meets your upper lip, making sure it's even. Then run a fine-tooth comb through your mustache from bottom to top, pulling away from your face as you go. Once you have your whole mustache in the comb, trim off any hairs that stick out. Doing so will make sure the hairs are all the same length and lay neatly on top of one another. Recomb your mustache from the top down to assess your work, and repeat the procedure if there are any stragglers. "It's best to be conservative the first time through, because you can always make it shorter but you can't make it longer," says Michael

Dwyer, a master barber at Vidal Sassoon in Manhattan.

If you still can't get your mustache to behave, buy some mustache wax. A little dab of the odorless, transparent cream will keep your hairs under control without being noticeable to eye or nose.

STOMACH CRAMPS

Q. I tend to get stomach cramps when I work out, and I've heard that drinking milk can cause the problem. Should I avoid milk before exercising?

—*E.S., Omaha, Nebraska*

A. It's unlikely that milk is causing your problem, says Nancy Clark, M.S., R.D., nutritionist at SportsMedicine Brookline and author of *Nancy Clark's Sports Nutrition Guidebook*. Milk would be to blame if you have a lactose intolerance or an allergic reaction to dairy products. Symptoms for both might include gassiness, bloating and diarrhea every time you drink milk or eat dairy products—whether you're exercising or not.

Stomach cramps are often caused by overeating or overexertion, while muscle cramps are usually caused by dehydration. To avoid the problem, keep your pre-workout meals small and fairly bland—eat toast, bananas, pretzels or dry cereal. Also, allow time for the food to digest: a half-hour for a small snack and up to four hours for a large meal. Drink plenty of water both before and during exercise.

BASHFUL BLADDER

Q. Since college, I've had a problem urinating in nervous situations and crowded public places. Even when I'm totally relaxed, my urine flow starts weak before getting stronger. It's become a terrible burden, and I need to know if something can be done. Can you recommend any medical procedures? Could this be totally mental?

—*J.L., Philadelphia, Pennsylvania*

A. You're suffering from what doctors call bashful bladder syndrome—a condition that we've all experienced at one time or another. What happens is that something makes you uneasy, and as a result, you involuntarily tense up the muscles that control the flow of urine out of your bladder. A lot of things can set this problem off—even just having the boss walk up to the next urinal. What complicates it all is worrying that it'll happen again. Then you get in a vicious cycle: Because you're worried, you tense up and can't pee. Because you can't pee, you're still worried, and so on.

It's not, in any case, a serious problem, since the pressure of the urine in your bladder will eventually overwhelm the muscles trying to hold it back. When the problem is at its worst, the easiest solution is to just wait for a stall in the bathroom. Funny how a little privacy makes all the difference.

You can overcome bashful bladder syndrome by learning how to consciously relax those muscles, say the experts. Practice stopping and starting your urine flow—in the privacy of your own bathroom, of course. If the problem is really a burden as you say, a psychiatrist can prescribe drugs to help relax those troublesome muscles.

REDNECK

Q. I get redness under my lip and on my neck from shaving. What can I do about it?

—*A.S., New York, New York*

A. Tell your children to stop sharpening their Crayolas with your razor. You don't have kids? Then the redness signals irritated skin, a common shaving hassle. John F. Romano, M.D., a dermatologist at The New York Hospital–Cornell Medical Center, offers these tips for a less grating shave.

■ If you use a blade, shower before you shave to soften your beard. When you are ready to shave, wet your face again with warm water and soap, then apply a shaving gel to seal in the moisture. Shave in the direction your beard grows and use short strokes. (A razor with a pivoting head will improve your control because it follows the curves.)

■ If you use an electric razor, shave before showering or washing your face. Because you'll be shaving a dry face, you don't want to wash off the natural oils that have accumulated on your skin overnight. They act as a protective barrier between your face and the electric razor. Prepping with a powder-based preshave helps, too. It's kinder to skin than one containing alcohol.

■ If you are still seeing red, see your doctor.

THE EXTRA STRETCH

Q. I've read that stretching after running can help keep my muscles more flexible. I stretch for at least ten minutes after every run, but my body never seems to get any more elastic. Am I doing something wrong, or was I just born stiff?
—*B.A., Mountain View, California*

A. Stretching after a run is only enough to counteract the muscle tightening that occurred during that run, says Pat Croce, physical conditioning coach for Philadelphia's 76ers and Flyers. If you want to really loosen up, you need to throw in some extra stretches at various times during the day. One of the easiest ways to work stretching into your schedule is to do a few minutes after you get up in the morning and a few more before going to bed. To avoid pulling a cold muscle, never bounce and always do at least two sets of each stretch—working up to 60 seconds per stretch.

WHERE DO I APPLY COLOGNE?

Q. What's the right amount of cologne to use, and where should I apply it?
—*A.M., Phoenix, Arizona*

A. The most common mistake men make with cologne is that they splash it on their faces, says Annette Green, director of the Fragrance Foundation in New York City. That not only dries out facial skin, because of the alcohol that's mixed in with the fragrance, but tends to result in too much of a good thing. You probably already know which of your coworkers are splashing on cologne; you can smell them coming around the corner.

Proper cologne use requires more subtlety. Put a few

drops on your fingertips, then dab lightly behind each ear with your fingers. If you want to live dangerously, rub a little on the center of your chest as well. Wash your hands with soap and warm water before going out—fragrant hand-shakes won't win you any points with business associates.

For the office, Green recommends lighter types of cologne, which are dominated by smells of citrus, mint or spice. Save heavier fragrances like musk, floral or woodsy scents for after hours. If you're not sure which is which, ask a salesperson at the fragrance counter.

Finally, even following these guidelines, you're going to run into problems if you use cologne with a different brand of scented shaving cream or after-shave. You'll end up with what fragrance-business people call "clashing scents."

CARCINOGENIC BOOZE

Q. I've heard that there's an ingredient in alcohol that may cause cancer. Is this true? Is it in all kinds of booze?

—*D.R., Versailles, Kentucky*

A. What you are referring to is not a single ingredient but a class of chemical compounds called congeners, which are produced during the fermentation process. Experts theorize that some of these may be carcinogenic, but they're not sure. It's known, for example, that heavy drinkers are more prone to mouth and throat cancer than the general population, but the precise element in liquor that causes cancer has not yet been identified. It's a complicated business: "Alcohol fermentation produces a whole host of by-products. The way in which these affect the body is not completely understood yet," admits John Brick, Ph.D., chief of research at Rutgers University.

What we do know is that congeners are more concentrated in darker liquors such as cognac, whiskey, dark beer and red wine than in clear ones such as vodka, gin, light beer and white wine. You might want to stick to the lighter ones if you're concerned. Even better, just drink less. "If you're having fewer than three drinks a day, your risk for cancer is probably not increased," says Dr. Brick.

READY-TO-USE EYEGLASSES OKAY?

Q. Lately, I've been having difficulty reading the fine type in some newspapers, so I've started wearing a pair of ready-to-use reading glasses I found at a pharmacy. Any danger in this?
—A.H., Palacios, Texas

A. Not as far as we can see. According to our experts, ready-to-use reading glasses are a safe and inexpensive way to correct a common kind of farsightedness known as presbyopia. It's caused when the lenses in our eyes begin to lose some of their elasticity, making it harder to focus on close-up objects. The problem usually becomes noticeable sometime around your fortieth birthday. Typically, you find yourself holding reading matter farther and farther away from your eyes. It's time for glasses when your arms aren't long enough to bring the type into focus.

To select the right pair of reading glasses, hold a newspaper at normal reading distance as you try on several pairs in ascending order of strength. There are 16 different levels of magnification, ranging from +1.00 (the weakest) to +4.00 (the strongest), and the glasses should be identified by these numbers on their hang tags. You'll know you've found the right pair when the print becomes clear and stays that way while you read for several minutes.

Should you begin to experience headaches or tired eyes while reading with your glasses, it's possible you have an underlying vision disorder that requires prescription lenses or treatment from an ophthalmologist. Ask your family doctor for a referral, or contact the National Society to Prevent Blindness at (800) 221-3004 for further information about choosing a qualified specialist.

TOO MANY HAMSTRING PULLS

Q. I'm a runner, and I seem to be getting more than my share of hamstring pulls. I've had several in each leg, usually during fairly short runs. I've started lifting weights to strengthen the backs of my legs, but that doesn't seem to have helped. What could be causing my problem?
—R.W., Morton, Illinois

A. You're probably overstriding, says John Marino, D.C., an avid runner and a member of the American Chiropractic Association's Council on Sports Injury and Physical Fitness. Increasing the length of your stride in an effort to run faster is one of the most common mistakes among runners, and it puts extra strain on the hamstrings. To run faster, increase the *speed* of your stride, not its length.

Weight training is a good idea, but be sure to work the quadriceps, the muscles in the fronts of your thighs, as well as the hamstrings. Strengthening only your hamstrings can create a strength imbalance that will leave you more suscep-tible to injury. Also, save your weight training for after your runs, because lifting can leave your muscles tight and prone to injury. In fact, it's best to run on a different day altogether. And always stretch immediately after lifting *or* running to keep your hamstrings flexible.

DANDRUFF SHAMPOO

Q. I have a slight problem with dandruff. A hairstylist told me that I should rub conditioner into my scalp, but it doesn't seem to be working. I shy away from dandruff shampoos because I've heard they will damage my hair. Any suggestions?

—N.C., Washington, D.C.

A. Rubbing the scalp vigorously, as your hairstylist recom-mends, may only loosen more dead skin cells, which is all dandruff really is anyway. It's also a mistake to use a mois-turizer or conditioner: The flaking and scaling may look as if it's caused by dry skin, but in fact, the opposite is true.

Which brings us to dandruff shampoos. These products contain ingredients that slow the rate at which scalp cells multiply and flake off. The shampoos have had to pass elabo-rate safety tests and won't damage your hair, says Guy Webster, M.D., Ph.D., assistant professor of dermatology at Jefferson Medical College of Thomas Jefferson University. Excessive flaking or itching that you can't get rid of with a dandruff shampoo indicates a more severe skin problem that requires a trip to the dermatologist.

LOW EJACULATE VOLUME

Q. I'm 38 years old, and over the past year I've noticed that my second and third ejaculations, even over several hours, produce very little semen. Although I had a vasectomy six years ago, I hadn't noticed any difference until now. Could that have anything to do with my problem? How can I restore the volume of my youth?

—C.O., Pasadena, California

A. Your vasectomy has nothing to do with it. The operation only blocks the release of sperm, which account for a very small percentage of the volume of the ejaculate.

As you get older, your body doesn't produce as much semen as it used to. So seeing some decline in the volume of your ejaculate is no surprise, especially if you're talking about multiple orgasms, says E. Douglas Whitehead, M.D., a director of the Association for Male Sexual Dysfunction.

There are no magic pills or foods that will increase your ejaculate volume. But the real question is: Why would you want to? Making too much of the statistical measurements of your performance won't make sex more enjoyable. In fact, it could make it worse. "If you keep telling yourself your performance is unsatisfactory, you can wind up talking yourself into not functioning at all," says Bill Young, director of the Masters and Johnson Institute in St. Louis. "Focus on the pleasure of sex. If you're doing it to keep score, you're going to lose."

BEST TEST

Q. Now that I'm 50, my doctor recommends that I be screened annually for prostate cancer. He mentioned several tests, but I would like to know which is most reliable.

—J.T., Newburyport, Massachusetts

A. You should get two tests at your screening: a PSA blood test and a digital rectal examination. The first is a measure of a blood chemical (prostate-specific antigen) that increases if the prostate enlarges. The second, a simple physical examination of the gland, allows your doctor to feel any irregularities in its size or shape. When done together, the tests are the most effective and reliable method for detecting prostate cancer, according to William Catalona, M.D., professor and chief of the division of urologic surgery at Washington University School of Medicine in St. Louis. The annual screenings should start at age 40 if a close relative had prostate cancer.

ARTHRITIC KNEES

Q. I am 32 years old and have arthritis in both of my knees. My doctor has suggested that I take two aspirin a day and avoid sports like tennis, basketball and running. Can you tell me what sports provide a good workout but are easy on the knees?
—M.B., New York, New York

A. Swimming is the exercise that's easiest on the knees. Just don't use a frog-leg kick, as this puts added stress on the injured cartilage in the joint. In deep water with a flotation device, you can also simulate the motions of running and biking without the negative effects of gravity.

Depending on how bad your problem is, bicycling on flat terrain, fitness walking and cross-country skiing may be safe as well. "Use your knees as a barometer. If they're painful after the exercise, you've gone too far," says Todd Molnar, physical medicine and rehabilitation specialist at the Southern California Orthopedic Center.

SAFE TIE FASHION

Q. Every time I buy new ties, styles change, and suddenly, I'm out of date. This year all my ties are too narrow. Is there a safe width I can buy that will always be in fashion?
—T.O., Bucksport, Maine

A. "Safe fashion is an oxymoron," chuckles Gerald Andersen, executive director of the Neckware Association of America, a guy who has been asked this question before. Moreover, ties don't suddenly get fat or thin, which leads us to surmise that the last time you bought ties was about five years ago, when they were 2 ½ inches wide. Today's ties are 3¾ inches across the base, and Anderson figures this width will be in style for at least two more years.

Fortunately, there's help for outdated neckware. Favorite old ties can easily be narrowed or widened (as long as there's enough material).

Send them to Tie Crafters, 116 East 27th Street, New York, NY 10016. The cost to alter a tie is $7.50; there's a four-tie minimum, and you need to add $3 for return shipping. Allow two weeks.

NIGHTMARES

Q. I have nightmares whenever I fall asleep on my back. This doesn't seem to happen if I sleep on my stomach. Is this common? What may be the reason for this?

—J.R., Columbia, Maryland

A. If you're a snorer, there could be a link between sleeping on your back and the nightmares you have. When you sleep belly-up, it's easy for your windpipe to narrow and the base of your tongue to fall back into your throat. That causes you to snore, interfering with your breathing. In many cases, the airway completely closes, and snorers actually stop breathing for five seconds to a minute or longer. This is a condition known as sleep apnea, and it affects about one-third of all loud snorers.

Interrupted breathing could easily trigger bad dreams, "particularly dreams of suffocating or being chased and out of breath," says Elliott Phillips, M.D., medical director of the North Valley Sleep Disorders Center in Mission Hills, California. The best way to tell if you have this problem is to ask your bed partner if you snore. Ask her to listen carefully to see if you stop breathing when you sleep. If you do, see a doctor. Severe sleep apnea may lead to high blood pressure, heart attack and stroke. But the problem is highly treatable.

ALLERGIC TO COMDOMS

Q. I think I'm allergic to latex condoms. I get a rash whenever I use one. I'm reluctant to use sheepskin condoms because I've heard they're not an effective barrier against diseases. Are there any options other than putting my sex life on hold?

—T.H., Lexington, Kentucky

A. Before you start apartment hunting in a monastery, test-drive different latex condoms. The manufacturing process differs enough from one to the next that it's possible you're just allergic to a single brand. Also, you could be reacting to the lubricant or spermicide on the condom you now use rather than to the latex itself, says Kenneth Goldberg, M.D., founder and director of the Male Health Center in Dallas. He suggests trying a nonlubricated condom.

If the rash persists, try a mild, over-the-counter steroid cream on your skin before donning the condom. You are wise to avoid using animal-skin condoms, which, as you pointed out, are not as effective a barrier against sexually transmitted diseases as latex ones are.

A DAY OFF

Q. I've been lifting weights for almost a year. My fitness instructor tells me I should be lifting every other day, but when I take two days off between workouts, I can do more repetitions or use heavier weights than if I rest for only one day. Is it okay to take an extra day off between workouts?

—W.P., Palm Bay, Florida

A. Another day of rest won't hurt. And if you've been training extra hard, you probably need it to give your muscles time to heal, says Wayne Campbell, M.S., of the Exercise Physiology Laboratory at Tufts University. He also says it's *not* a good idea to knock yourself out at every single workout. Research shows that consistently pushing yourself to your limit won't build you up any faster. Instead, it will only increase your risk of injury.

A safer and more effective lifting routine is to go for the really big weights no more than once a week. Balance this heavy day with lighter workouts the rest of the week. "That way, you'll maximize your training, minimize your risk of injury and continue to improve," says Campbell.

A suggested schedule: On Monday and Wednesday, use weights that are light enough for you to do 8 to 12 repetitions in each of three sets. (You should be able to recover from this workout with a single day off.) On Friday, go for the heavy weights that make you reach fatigue between the sixth and eighth repetitions of each set. Take weekends off.

To further protect your muscles from tightness and soreness, be sure to stretch every day.

AVOID WRINKLES

Q. I'm 38 years old, and I'm one of those men who are trying to slow down facial wrinkling. Okay, so I'm a little vain. But tell me, does regular use of a moisturizer put the brakes on the wrinkling process? And will the use of only plain soap and water give me more wrinkles?

—W.N., Rochester, New York

A. To avoid wrinkled skin, first and foremost, stay out of the sun. Ultraviolet rays, not soap and water, are the culprits, says dermatologist Jonathan S. Weiss, M.D., a clinical assistant professor at Emory University School of Medicine.

Using moisturizers daily won't slow down the wrinkling process, but it will help disguise those crow's-feet by hydrating the skin. Dry skin, often brought on by washing with plain soap and water, makes wrinkles stand out. Switch to a moisturizing soap such as Dove or Basis for extra-dry skin, or try a soap-free cleanser such as Cetaphil.

A good defense against wrinkles, suggests Dr. Weiss, is a daily application of a fragrance-free sunscreen containing moisturizer in place of your after-shave. And if you plan to be outdoors for a long time, cover your skin with sunscreen with a sun protection factor (SPF) of at least 15.

POST-SEX ACHE

Q. Sometimes right after sex, I get an ache in my testicles. What could be causing the problem?

—R.L., Reno, Nevada

A. Post-ejaculatory pain can be caused by spasms of the pelvic muscles, a result of straining too hard during sex. To ease the soreness, try taking a hot bath. If the pain persists, chances are you've got a urinary infection. The infection could be as far up as your prostate, says Dr. Goldberg. Visit your doctor; he will probably conduct a urinalysis and a prostate exam. If you have an infection, your doctor will most likely treat it with antibiotics.

Index